DISCARDED

CALMER
WATERS

*The Caregiver's
Journey Through
Alzheimer's and
Dementia*

YUMA COUNTY
LIBRARY DISTRICT
2951 S. 21st Dr. Yuma, AZ 85364
(928) 782-1871
www.yumalibrary.org

BARBRA COHN

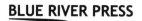

BLUE RIVER PRESS

Indianapolis, Indiana

Calmer Waters: The Caregiver's Journey Through Alzheimer's and Dementia

Copyright © 2016 Barbra Cohn

Published by Blue River Press
Indianapolis, Indiana
www.brpressbooks.com

Distributed by Cardinal Publishers Group
Tom Doherty Company, Inc.
www.cardinalpub.com

All rights reserved under International and
Pan-American Copyright Conventions.

No part of this book may be reproduced, stored in a database
or other retrieval system, or transmitted in any form, by any
means, including mechanical, photocopy, recording or otherwise,
without the prior written permission of the publisher.

ISBN: 978-1-68157-014-3

Author: Barbra Cohn
Editor: Morgan Sears
Interior Design: Dave Reed
Cover Design: David Miles
Cover Photo: Shutterstock_53882188

Published: 2016

Printed in the United States of America

The contents of this work are designed to provide helpful information
on the subjects discussed. References are provided for informational
purposes only and do not constitute endorsement of any websites or
other sources. This book is not intended as a substitute for the medical
advice of physicians. The publisher nor the author shall be liable for any
damages arising herefrom.

In Memory of Morris

For Ari, Bobette, and Hillary,
and the millions of sons, daughters,
spouses, and family members
who have lost their loved ones to
Alzheimer's Disease

CALMER WATERS

The Caregiver's Journey through Alzheimer's and Dementia

Part Four - *When Caregiving Ends*

Preface

After my husband had a heart attack in 1994, a friend told him that he appeared to have one foot in heaven. Morris was more focused on the celestial world and less engaged in his life on earth. He hibernated in his home office, and spent just a handful of hours at his business office each week. He watched too much television, and filled much of his day meditating. His greatest joy was participating in spiritual singing groups (kirtans) once a month in Boulder or Denver.

As Morris became disinterested in work and more forgetful and irritable, I urged him to see a neurologist. He was eventually diagnosed with younger-onset Alzheimer's disease, and I spent a decade caring for him before he died in the summer of 2010. Now that he has passed away, I've created lemonade out of lemons in order to help other caregivers and family members.

During his downward spiral, Morris developed the fragile demeanor of other Alzheimer's and dementia patients who do seem to have one foot in heaven; in a world that is easier to navigate than the temporal world that requires full cognition and social interaction. Sometimes while I drove him around town, he'd be alert one moment and then suddenly his head would drop onto his chest. Minutes later, he'd open his eyes and enjoy the music playing on the radio, as if no time had passed.

Individuals with dementia can be listening to the birds chirping, a TV show, or to a caregiver's encouraging words and then their memory jolts, and their attention is suddenly drawn inward or outward. Just hearing a character on the television refer to a son or daughter, a dog, or cupcake can trigger a cascade of behaviors that might range from the hilarious to frenetic. There is often no rhyme or reason for certain behaviors or stories told by a person with dementia. We have no way of knowing what type of thinking goes on in the dementia brain, but sometimes it seems that the person's consciousness hovers between earth and heaven. Sometimes it even appears that a person with dementia is communicating with deceased loved ones who are, of course, invisible to the casual observer.

Calmer Waters: The Caregiver's Journey through Alzheimer's and Dementia offers a glimpse into my family's journey. But even more importantly, it offers wisdom and tools and techniques that can help you feel happier, healthier and more relaxed, have more energy and time for yourself, sleep better, and ultimately experience inner peace. An added bonus is that it includes twenty healing modalities that help ease stress and anxiety in both caregivers and those with memory loss. When the caregiver engages the memory-impaired individual in one of these modalities a stronger connection is forged between the two care partners, and then they both feel better.

Caregivers typically feel stressed, tired, and worried. When you spend hours each day feeding, dressing, and toileting a loved one, you have little time to take care of your own needs. You might feel a range of emotions including resentful, lonely, unhappy, depressed … and guilty. And if you have to get up during the night to help your care partner with toileting, wandering, or anxiety, you might not have the energy to get through the day without the aid of too many cups of coffee. Stress, lack of sleep, and worry can take a huge toll on a caregiver's health, which is what inspired me to write this book.

I started writing *Calmer Waters* when Morris was in mid-stage Alzheimer's disease. I had to put it on the back burner as my caregiving demands increased. And, as the disease progressed, the focus of the book shifted. It developed into something more than I envisioned each time I found a person who enthusiastically contributed an essay or article. I invited other families to contribute to the book because as the saying goes, "Once you've seen one Alzheimer's patient, you've seen one." And once you've entered the world of one family coping with this disease, you've entered a realm in which all members have a unique style of maintaining sanity and dignity in a universe that has gone awry.

I've learned a tremendous amount about compassion, love, kindness, suffering, grief, loss, joy, and strength as a caregiver and from the families and professionals who contributed to *Calmer Waters*. They helped me to deeply understand what it means to be a care partner on a long, painful journey, and how to strive to maintain love and compassion for all sentient beings.

I will be forever grateful to them for openly sharing their personal stories, wisdom, and guidance.

If this book helps uplift your family and strengthens your coping skills, it will have fulfilled its purpose. And if every reader gains one bit of wisdom or insight into the miraculous self-discovery that you are forced to embark upon through your selfless work, the contributors to *Calmer Waters* can rejoice in knowing they have aided and soothed a caregiver, as well as the person you so lovingly and generously care for. Stay strong.

Blessings,

Barbra Cohn

Acknowledgements

There are so many people to thank for helping my family and me as we journeyed on a path that too many people are forced to take. And there are many people to thank for supporting me in the writing of this book.

First, thank you to my family and friends for their support, especially Bobette Cohn, Ari and his wife Ronit Cohn, and Hillary and her husband Daniel Aizenman for always being there for their father (and father-in-law) and me with love and tenderness; to my parents Irving and Thelma Levine who opened their hearts and ears with compassion, love, and support; and to the wonderful friends who provided the support and love so vital during a decade-long catastrophic illness: Randy and Michael Faulkner, Anand Grace, Harley Fisher, Judith Landsman, Steve Milligan, Kay and Keith Puckett, Steve Rosen, Tom Mahowald, Mary Stevenson, Bob Wampler, and our beloved Tuesday lunch group. A special thank you to Michelle Pelc and Katie Stefanski who devoted loving care to Morris with ingenuity, grace, and humor.

Thank you to the Alzheimer's Association, and especially to the Denver younger-onset support group. The support group that Morris and I attended for several years formed a formidable bond that continues even after our spouses, and mothers, and fathers succumbed to Alzheimer's disease. Professionals at the Denver Alzheimer's Association welcomed me with open arms when I was desperately in need of comfort and information. A special thanks to Shelley Karp, Mattye Pollard-Cole, Graham Kolb, Deb Wells, Diane Scholl, Judy Lyons, Marcia Reish, Ron Jepson, Phyllis Willmoth, Nancy Hahn, Stacey Remer, Sara Spaulding, and Linda Mitchell.

Thank you to the incredible staff at Juniper Village, Balfour Senior Living, and TRU Care Community, formerly called Boulder and Broomfield County Hospice. A very special thanks to our inimitable doctor Julie Carpenter, MD, and to Andrew Bunin, MA, LSW. You all provided me with a guiding light while I struggled to walk through a black hole.

Thank you to my wonderful two writing groups. My daytime group: Joan Knaub, Sue McMillan, Barbara Sable, Antoinette Rose, and Rose Marie Khubchandani, who provided encouragement, suggestions, and open hearts. Thank you to my evening group: Barbara Foster, Rohini Grace, Kathy Hunter, Laura Guerra Perez, and Nancy Kirkendall, who listened carefully, commented gently, and provided food, comfort, good times, and cherished friendship. Thank you to Renay Oshop for book publishing advice, to my editors Ellen Burkett and Morgan Sears, and to the team at Cardinal Publishing Group.

I am forever grateful to Sri Sai Kaleshwar Swami, Karunamayi, and Rabbi Marc Soloway for the spiritual guidance and wisdom that comforted Morris' soul and sustained mine. And to John Doyle for being my rock, and providing me with love, companionship, and nourishment for my body and soul.

* * *

Creating a Platform of Strength

Resources

Three web sites provide opportunities for caregivers to set up support networks of friends and family.

Lotsa Helping Hands™, lotsahelpinghands.com, is a wonderful tool to help caregivers network with a community established online that helps coordinate support during times of crisis and caregiver burnout. For instance, you're taking care of your mother at home, you work a part-time job out of the house, and you have two teenagers to care for. You're exhausted! Create a community of support on Lotsa Helping Hands™ to help you get your mother to a doctor's appointment, have a meal delivered, get respite care a couple hours a day, or whatever else you need. It's very doable, and you can do it from anywhere you live in the world.

Care Circles, www.carecircle.com. A Care Circle program is a website that you can purchase and set up in about ten minutes to let friends and family know what kind of support you need as a caregiver. Included is a private website that has multiple features including a Home page, a Guest Book where visitors can leave messages, a Photo Gallery, and a Calendar where friends can volunteer to deliver meals, take the person you are caring for to an appointment, or provide respite care or housekeeping. You can add pages and title them anyway you choose. You also get a Library that contains ways to assess your needs, involve others, and ideas for advertising your site.

CaringBridge, www.caringbridge.org, provides you with the tools to set up a free website to share health updates, videos, and photos with family and friends who want to help. It is especially useful during a crisis or for end-of-life assistance with the coordination of tasks such as delivering meals, providing childcare, arranging transportation, emotional support, and other organizational help.

Introduction

There were several indications that something was wrong with my husband two years before he was diagnosed. This tall, good-looking man, a graduate of the Wharton School of Business at the University of Pennsylvania, was having trouble calculating how much tip to leave a waitress. When we went to Spain for our twenty-fifth anniversary, Morris couldn't figure out how much money the hotel would cost in dollars. This man, who once memorized train and airplane schedules without even trying, followed me around the city like a puppy dog as we boarded a subway or bus en route to tourist attractions.

That following fall — our daughter's last year in high school — Morris couldn't give directions to her friend who was taking the SAT at the high school he had attended in Denver. I got out the map to help him, but he couldn't read the map. That was the moment I knew something was very wrong. When he left for a road trip to California with our son and forgot his suitcase, I sat on the stairs and cried. I couldn't deny it any longer. I had a strong suspicion that Morris had Alzheimer's disease, and although I pleaded with him for two years to see a neurologist, he refused.

Finally, he agreed. The doctor (I'll call her "Dr. Fitzgerald") asked Morris why he had come in. "My wife thinks I might have Alzheimer's disease," he said.

"You wouldn't be able to drive here yourself if you had Alzheimer's," she replied.

Nonetheless, Dr. Fitzgerald gave Morris the Mini-Mental State Exam (MMSE, a thirty point questionnaire used to screen cognitive impairment), asking questions such as, "What are the year, season, date, day, and month?" and progressing to more difficult questions that included counting backward from one hundred by serial sevens. I don't know about you, but I'd probably be slow on the draw to count backward by sevens. At least I'd have to stop and think about it before responding. Morris botched up that question, and he wasn't able to draw the face of a clock either. The concept of time was already an elusive abstraction.

Dr. Fitzgerald ordered a blood work-up to rule out an organic problem such as hypoactive thyroid—which can cause memory problems—and an MRI scan (magnetic resonance imaging) to rule out a brain tumor. To tell you the truth, I was hoping for a brain tumor because at least you can take the bull by the horns and really go at the darn thing with radiation and a scalpel. Well, there was no brain tumor and his blood panel looked just fine.

A week later, just as we were investigating the cost of long-term health insurance, Dr. Fitzgerald called to ask Morris to bring in his wife to the follow-up appointment. I'm sorry to say that one of the biggest mistakes I've ever made was to schedule that appointment without first buying long-term care insurance. Once you get a diagnosis such as Alzheimer's, there's no way you're going to qualify for long-term care insurance, which could potentially save a family thousands of dollars in catastrophic health care costs.

In the early afternoon of January 3, 2001, Morris and I sat in a dimly lit exam room on wooden frame chairs with hunter green cushions on the seat and back. He wore a sweater woven from various shades of blue and gray that highlighted his eyes. We waited for the doctor to knock on the door, the way they usually do. Morris didn't appear nervous; probably because he didn't think there was anything wrong with him. But my stomach was wound tight from anxiety and my lungs were working hard to expel phlegm. It didn't help that the stale re-circulated air had a metallic odor of fear that was probably generated by patients who had received bad news.

Dr. Fitzgerald finally came in and sat on Morris's left. She had cropped hair and spoke in a blunt, choppy cadence that matched her no-nonsense appearance. Without much of an introduction, the doctor asked me a few questions about Morris, speaking as if he were invisible.

"How is his driving?" she asked.

"He tends to get lost driving in familiar neighborhoods," I responded, noting the twitch in Morris's right cheek. I felt my lungs squeeze, and a high-pitched wheeze escaped from my chest.

"Here is the Mini-Mental State Exam Morris took the last time we met."

His drawing of a house looked like a dilapidated mine shaft. Without waiting for a response, Dr. Fitzgerald turned to Morris and said, "You have Alzheimer's disease."

Morris froze and his face turned white, while I burst out crying. I blubbered things like "I already have a lot of stress," and "I'm dealing with another health crisis."

Looking back, I can't imagine what kind of stress I was dealing with that measured anywhere close to being a caregiver for someone with Alzheimer's disease. And health crisis? Yeah, I had a bad case of bronchitis and asthma at the time. But an acute infection is easily remedied with antibiotics, a steroid inhaler, chicken soup, and rest. You address it, take care of it, and get over it. With an Alzheimer's diagnosis, if you are the family member, you listen in disbelief, go through various stages of grief (which manage to reappear on a continuous basis throughout the entire illness), and struggle with chronic stress for years. If you are the patient, you listen in disbelief, go through a grieving process, and embark on a dark, lonely journey, which finally ends after you've lost your mind and your life.

"What is the prognosis?" I managed to ask.

"He won't be able to drive in a few years, and I'm sorry, but there's not much we can do. I'm sorry." Those were the only kind words we ever heard from that doctor. She offered no hope or encouragement, other than mumbling that we should stop by her other office to pick up some literature about local support groups.

Morris and I managed to walk out the front door without breaking down. We stopped for gas on the way home, and I helped him put the credit card in the slot and the nozzle in the tank. We didn't speak, but the shock of a terminal diagnosis sent waves of terror throughout my body. And although Morris didn't utter a word, I felt the tension bounce off his skin like static in a dry room. Although I'm quite certain he didn't understand the full meaning of what it would be like to endure the rest of his life with this dreadful disease, on some level he knew that life would never again be light and easy.

Once we were inside the safety net of our home, we fell into each other's arms and cried. And I promised to help him get well. I promised the moon and the stars ... if only he'd get well.

I had to leave almost immediately for my own doctor's appointment, where I collapsed and cried that my husband had just been diagnosed with Alzheimer's. The doctor was sympathetic and concerned that I had pneumonia, and sent me to the hospital for a chest x-ray. I called Morris, told him I'd be late, and stopped for antibiotics on the way home. Entering our home was the beginning of a long, painful course in developing survival skills for living in a world turned upside down. The years I cared for Morris were a test of learning how to hide behind a veil of fear and tears . . . a test of strength, patience, and kindness. I've realized that this test was the most important spiritual challenge of my life.

I'm pretty confident that I will never again have to cope with another challenge of this magnitude. People in my family will get sick and we'll have new mountains to climb, roadblocks to avoid, and incomprehensible puzzles to figure out. My father died one year before Morris did, and eventually I'll have to bury my mother and face my own mortality. But nothing will ever compare to the ongoing pain of watching the person I vowed to share my life with (including the good times and bad) steadily decline from an intelligent man to a person who was dependent on me for placing all his meals in front of him, directing him to the water faucet, changing the TV channels, dialing his friends, chauffeuring him around town, and so much more. I watched him turn into a child who was unable to sustain an interesting conversation and whose greatest daily joy was watching crime shows and action movies. Although life is full of surprises, as I well know, I think that nothing will ever again grind my nerves and chip away my thin veneer of patience and strength as did caring for a person with Alzheimer's.

Did I enjoy being a caregiver? Honestly, no. Some individuals find that caring for a loved one deepens their love for that person and uplifts them spiritually. Although I gained little pleasure from my role, I've grown tremendously as a human being and I learned that it is possible to strengthen one's spiritual connection through self-sacrifice.

I also realized that caring for Morris was my spiritual challenge, so it was up to me to create joy and learn everything I could from caring for a sweet soul who became totally centered in his heart instead of his mind … for a man who was transformed from my partner into someone I didn't always recognize. Someone who would morph into a tender, young boy, an angry, rebellious teen or a helpless old man.

People would say to me, "I could never do what you're doing" or "You're an angel." Believe me, I'm no angel and I had no intention of becoming a martyr, but I was committed to take care of Morris until I was no longer able to. And so, I listened to the experts and to my therapist insist that I had to take care of myself. I made sure I had time to nurture my soul and do some of the things I love, which included my passion – dancing. When it became too difficult for me to take care of Morris on my own, I hired caregivers. And when I felt myself breaking in pieces little by little, when I realized caring for him would harm my health, I placed Morris in a memory care home. I decided early on that I wasn't going to let this disease ruin my life.

Morris passed away the end of August 2010. There was a nest of birds outside his window, and for two weeks I watched the mother bird bring food to her babies. Morris didn't see them, but he heard the joyful chirping of new life and the excited anticipation that accompanies it. The chicks left the nest moments after Morris took his last breath. It was a bright, clear, breezy day, and the wind stood still just long enough for the birds to show Morris the way home.

Part One

✕

The Spirituality
of Caregiving

1

My Life Wasn't Supposed to
Turn Out This Way

Barbra and Morris Cohn

At time of Morris's diagnosis:
Morris — sixty years old
Barbra — forty-eight years old
Children — Bobette - thirty-eight,
Ari - twenty-one,
Hillary - eighteen

> "Life's under no obligation to give us what we expect."
> – Margaret Mitchell

* * *

"My life wasn't supposed to turn out this way," I choked through tears, as I relayed Morris's diagnosis on the phone to my parents.

It's not as though I hadn't dealt with illness or death before, but I had always felt that my life was charmed. I lived in beautiful Boulder, Colorado, with a loving, devoted husband and two of our fabulous children, had wonderful friends, an interesting career as a health writer, a wealth of activities — hiking, playing the piano, dancing, meditating — and plenty of other interests to keep me busy and fulfilled. I was happy. So when the traumas piled up like fresh blankets of snow covering the dirty ones, I began to feel akin to Job.

Shortly after my husband was diagnosed with Alzheimer's disease, our house was flooded by a leaky farmer's ditch. Two years later it flooded again, and this time I did what I should have done in the first place. I had the entire basement floor jack hammered, so that a French drain and sump pump could be installed. The entire contents of Morris's home office — which included a library containing about two thousand books — a bedroom, a den, bathroom, and storage room had to be carried upstairs to the living and dining rooms and garage, where it remained for several months. Not an easy thing for anyone, but for someone already disoriented by Alzheimer's disease, it was disruptive and mind boggling, to say the least. Then, as I was trying to cope with the pain of losing the man I had married, our beloved Scottish terrier died from bladder cancer. And finally, because of financial woes, we were forced to sell the house we had built and raised our children in.

The year preceding the move was very difficult. We averaged three showings a week, and cleaning the house and planning an outing with my husband each time was stressful and strenuous. But I miraculously survived without succumbing to as much as a single cold. All the while, not only did I manage things efficiently, I felt like "superwoman." I was able to move large heavy items that normally a woman my size wouldn't be able to move without help. I lost my footing once, dropped a box of books, and landed on concrete. I got up immediately, but my skinned and bruised knee hurt for a month. That didn't stop me from doing anything that I wanted or needed to do.

That mishap metaphorically captures the essence of the ten-year Alzheimer's journey our family took. Although it was a time of profound, deeply felt loss, I realized that I had a lot to be grateful for, and that things could always get worse. For the most part, I didn't allow myself to submit to feeling like a victim, feeling sorry for myself, or wanting pity. For the longest time, I lived behind a persona of forced cheerfulness because I didn't want anyone to know that my private world was being deconstructed bit by bit. I went through bouts of depression and grieving periods. But for the most part, I was able to maintain a positive attitude, hoping for a medical miracle. Until the day we placed Morris in a memory care home, there was always one more supplement to take, one more healer to visit, one more guru to lead us on the road to recovery.

When Morris was diagnosed, I was hopeful that we would be blessed with a medical miracle or one of divine intervention. In fact, I was so sure that he would be "cured" that one of the reasons I refrained from telling people about his condition was I thought he'd get well; so why bother telling anyone about it? We also agreed not to share the information — outside of our family and very close friends — because of the stigma attached to Alzheimer's disease. We were embarrassed. What would people think about someone who developed Alzheimer's after spending half of his life meditating in order to develop his consciousness?

Also, I didn't want people scrutinizing Morris's every word and action. People tend to treat those with serious chronic diseases differently. They shy away from that person as though he or she is contagious. We were pretty lucky as far as friends go. Most of them supported us throughout the challenging years. Some fell by the wayside, as is often the case when someone receives a dreadful diagnosis. It hurt, but I understand that some people don't have the emotional or psychological strength, skills, or life experience for facing problems of this magnitude. I have heard from others, though, that their friends abandoned them completely — and it's very painful to try to stay afloat in the midst of a tsunami when all support is taken away.

I was philosophical about our situation because of my spiritual experience and practice. In fact, I surprised myself when I had the epiphany that, although it's not something I would ever have chosen, if I had never experienced the tragedy of my husband's disease and its effect on our family, I wouldn't be the person I am today. Who is that person? I always thought of myself as being mature, kind, sincere, and compassionate, but when I think back to when Morris was first diagnosed, I realize how much I've developed as a human being. That may sound trite, but it's actually profound when I measure the growth in relation to my perspective of where I was before and where I am now — no matter how unscientific or subjective the measurement is.

I once believed that I would skate through life by occasionally tripping over cracks and crevices, but avoiding collisions with icebergs. I now know that no one escapes from this life without facing at least one life-transforming challenge, no matter the form it comes in. And no matter how fervently mystics proclaim that life is bliss and that we should never have to suffer, I believe that living a blissful life is an admirable goal for all human beings and a definite possibility for a few, but there is a lot of suffering we inevitably endure during a lifetime. The key to rising above it is to understand that even though you can't always control what happens to you, you can control how you respond.

Thankfully, the techniques and healing modalities compassion-ately offered by healers and spiritual leaders, and the healing wisdom shared by caregivers, can make the Alzheimer's journey less painful and transform it into a profound spiritual experience. I continually remind myself of Sri Sai Kaleshwar Swami's favorite adage, "Life is short, make it sweet." I've learned that in this life we need to expect the unexpected, and that the basis of creating a meaningful life begins with treating others as we'd like to be treated, with kindness and compassion and without judgment.

2

Caregiving from a Spiritual Perspective

Our beliefs about spirituality, religion, and personal philosophy greatly affect how we care for others. Those beliefs and how we put them into action equally have a profound effect on our health. This chapter sets the groundwork for care partners (the caregiver and the person being cared for) to connect on a spiritual level and how to create an environment that provides that opportunity.

"We could never learn to be brave and patient
if there were only joy in the world."
– Helen Keller

Spirituality is a personal connection that one feels with God, a higher purpose, a higher being, nature, or with one's self — or that part of yourself referred to as the soul. Spirituality is very individualized and doesn't require a practice or adherence to a set of beliefs. Many people express their spirituality through a philosophy, a particular lifestyle, a religion, or a continual search for meaning and purpose in life. Some people fulfill a spiritual need by seeking harmony with nature, music, or art. Some attain their spiritual aspirations through meditation and yoga.

Living a spiritual life incorporates nurturing humanistic qualities such as compassion, love, tolerance, forgiveness, patience, and tranquility, and the commitment to help others. Caregiving from a spiritual perspective — regardless of the form it takes — is an effective way of managing some of the stress and emotional issues that accompany caring for someone with dementia. Anger is one of the emotions that can arise in dementia caregiving. Researchers have found that people who care for dementia patients are angrier than non-caregivers, with forty percent of them irritable some or most of the time. This isn't surprising, especially when a caregiver might be caring for someone who repeats the same question repeatedly, refuses to eat what you've prepared for dinner, paces around the room one hundred times per hour, or has his or her days and nights reversed.

But relating on the level of spirit, while knowing that the person with Alzheimer's will never recover, allows for communication that transcends language. It supports a loving connection that can diminish anger, irritation, and resentment towards the patient, allowing the caregiver to ease the negative mind chatter, psychological distress, and toxic emotions that can take a toll on physical health.

A relationship rooted in spirituality

It was natural, albeit not easy, for me to care for Morris from a spiritual perspective because our relationship was based on our spiritual philosophy, practice, and way of life. I have always felt a holy presence in my life. We are here for a short time and it's our responsibility to help heal the world and each other, and to help each other achieve our potential. I had an unusually rich early childhood and plenty of opportunity to put that philosophy into action.

I grew up in a three-family house with an aunt, uncle, and cousin who lived on the bottom floor, my Orthodox Jewish grandparents on the middle floor, and my nuclear family on the top floor. While we lived above my grandparents, I wasn't allowed to draw or cut paper on Saturdays—Shabbat—and I often watched my grandfather put on teffillin (tiny boxes that contain holy scrolls) every morning and daven (pray). Jewish holidays were gargantuan, rowdy events in which my four aunts and their husbands and children, and two uncles and their wives and children, sat at my grandparents' large dining room table feasting on matzoh ball soup, noodle and potato kugels, chicken, brisket, and tzimmes (a sweet dish made with carrots, prunes, and potatoes).

When I was eight years old, my parents, younger brother, and I moved to the country. I attended religious school three times a week until I became a Bat Mitzvah. I loved listening to Rabbi Jerome Malino lecture about the three tenets of Judaism: Israel, Torah, and God. When I was nineteen years old, I spent the summer in the Negev on a kibbutz — a collective farm or community in modern Israel where everyone works and lives together. This is where I had my first "spiritual" experience of a divine presence.

At the kibbutz I was assigned to pick peaches and apricots in the orchard. Because the temperature got up to 110 degrees by midday, we awoke at 4 a.m. so we could finish working by noon. The air was so thin and dry that water droplets evaporated within minutes. Concrete and asphalt surfaces were so hot that blisters erupted on the soles of your feet, if you were crazy enough to walk barefoot. Thankfully, the lacy canopy of leaves offered a bit of protection from the relentless sun.

I rarely spoke while I picked the giant fuzzy jewels and was careful to gently place each one inside a woven basket. I preferred my own thoughts to the idle gossip that buzzed in and out of the tree branches. At 8 a.m. we'd break for an Israeli salad of tomatoes, cucumber, bell peppers, hard-boiled eggs, and bread, which was served in a makeshift hut covered by a tin roof.

One afternoon, instead of sleeping away the hottest hours of the day and then swimming in the pool before dinner, I wandered into the desert, away from the kibbutz. I came to a cluster of date trees and watched the orange and pink ribbons of light blaze across the sky as the sun made its descent. Except for a few birds that swooped through the trees, everything was perfectly quiet and peaceful. The silence was deep and profound, and in that moment my awareness was acute. I felt connected to every grain of sand, pebble, and rock. Images of faces in the rocks seemed to speak to me. I felt connected to a higher intelligence—to God, to a Divine Being—that underlies all creation.

This experience opened my consciousness and curiosity. Soon afterwards I became a vegetarian because I had the realization that I didn't need to eat an animal whose life had to be sacrificed in order for me to live. When I returned to the U.S., I learned how to meditate and ended up switching my college major from biology to religious studies. I needed to know what inspired people to seek God. What were their spiritual practices and where did they originate? What is it that moves people to pray together to a divine being or god? What are the outcomes? Why is so much violence perpetuated as a consequence of the desire to be holy?

My quest brought me to Boulder — which I had heard was a New Age Mecca — and to Morris.

The first time I met Morris

I waited until the crowd thinned and approached the stage where Morris had just given an introductory lecture on Transcendental Meditation™. It was 1972, and I was nineteen years old with waist-length, lustrous, chestnut hair scented from lemon shampoo. I wore patched jeans, an inside-out baby blue sweatshirt, and knee-high, lace-up moccasins. I had fallen in love with Transcendental Meditation (TM), which I learned several months before transferring as a second semester student to the University of Colorado in Boulder. The semester had just begun and I didn't have any friends. I was lonely for the first time in my life. So I went to the TM lecture on campus with high hopes of connecting with the meditating community.

Morris was a celebrated TM teacher who had just returned from a course taught by Maharishi Mahesh Yogi in La Antilla, Spain. He spent a month there meditating and listening to lectures about the Vedas (Sanskrit holy books), and he was beaming like a child who was about to share his magic tricks with a roomful of thrill-seekers. He appeared goofy with his wire-rimmed glasses, camel corduroy jacket (patched at the elbows), reddish moustache, and medium-length curly brown hair. The audience, filled with college students and Boulderites, loved it when he punctuated his paragraphs with a giggle.

Morris spoke about the benefits of diving deep into pure consciousness with the aid of a mantra (a sound that has beneficial effects on the physiology), and emerging energized and relaxed. The people seemed entranced by the message of attaining a state of peacefulness and living a more successful, happier life. Cindy, another teacher, took the stage when Morris was finished talking. She told the group about the preparatory lecture for those interested in learning TM. Afterwards, I approached the stage where Morris and I exchanged our first words. He asked me to help with the meditation initiations on the weekend and I agreed.

That was the beginning of a friendship—which was, more or less, like a teacher-student relationship—that lasted several years before we became romantically involved. Our relationship took root in the spiritual practice we shared, and grew steadily as we eventually taught TM together and went to meditation retreats. No matter what happened throughout the years, whether we saw eye-to-eye on various issues or disagreed, we shared the same spiritual values and practice that nourished our souls.

So when it came time for me to serve Morris as a spiritual caregiver, I understood that the job would require me to fall back into the teacher-student relationship where we began our journey together. I was Morris's caregiver, but he was again my teacher, making me more aware of my words, my actions, and my thoughts, than ever before. Sometimes I rose to the occasion, and sometimes I failed to listen and act with compassion. It was a challenge to care for him and stay grounded in my spirituality. But I tried, and I continue to try to forgive myself for the times that I failed.

The impact of religion and spirituality on health

Researchers at the Mayo Clinic reviewed studies that examined the association between religious involvement and spirituality with physical and mental health, health-related quality of life, and other health outcomes. In their published report, *Religious Involvement, Spirituality, and Medicine: Implications for Clinical Practice*, the authors noted that "most studies have shown that religious involvement and spirituality are associated with better health outcomes, including greater longevity, coping skills, and health-related quality of life (even during terminal illness) and less anxiety, depression, and suicide."

The report says that religious and spiritual practices such as meditation, prayer, and worship engender positive emotions such as hope, love, contentment, and forgiveness, and limit negative emotions such as hostility. These positive emotions have a physiological component. They help decrease activation of the sympathetic branch of the autonomic nervous system and the hypothalamic-pituitary-adrenal axis, which leads to a decrease in the release of stress hormones such as norepinephrine and cortisol. The correlating physiological response is lowered blood pressure, heart rate, and oxygen consumption, and leads to a stronger immune system. The correlating psychological effect is less anxiety and more happiness.

Enhancing the spiritual connection between care partners

As a panel member of the eighteenth annual Living With Grief® Program, Hospice Foundation of America (April 13, 2011, Washington, DC) Carolyn Jacobs, PhD, dean, professor, and director of the Contemplative Clinical Practice Advanced Certificate Program at the Smith College School for Social Work, spoke on the topic of spirituality and end-of-life care. When people are ill, or face a terminal disease, they usually become introspective, and spirituality often comes into play, said Dr. Jacobs. A search for something more transcendent than how they have lived their life is integral to the end of life; an expression of spirituality is a way of healing and asking for forgiveness. Dying individuals have a need to define a sense of meaning to their life and to find hope beyond the grave. Spiritual experience helps the patient deal with the pain of their situation or accept it more easily. There is also an urgent need for the dying or sick individual's family to assure him or her that they will carry on sacred family traditions, says Jacobs. Ultimately, the person's legacy is built from the relationships that have been nurtured over the course of a lifetime. If those relationships were fraught with pain and bitterness, the end-of-life struggle can be more painful, added Dr. Jacobs.

When a person with dementia approaches the end of life, he or she is usually unable to speak, so the person's spirituality or expression of it might not be apparent at all to a caregiver or other observer. But caregivers are sometimes surprised by a special presence, a glow, and the ability to radiate love even more than when the person with dementia was healthy.

This was the case with Morris. As his disease progressed, he became more and more heart centered. Because his brain cells were dying from the build-up of amyloid plaques and neurofibrillary tangles — the hallmarks of Alzheimer's disease — he lost his short-term memory, critical thinking skills, ability to rationalize, spatial awareness, and speech. He never stopped recognizing his close family members or friends, however, which seems to be typical of younger-onset Alzheimer's disease patients as opposed to older folks who get Alzheimer's in their seventies, eighties, and nineties. These older individuals tend to survive longer and often reach a vegetative state where they are unable to recognize their closest relatives. But Morris knew me and our children up until the moment he died.

One way to make a spiritual connection

I try to adhere to Martin Buber's philosophy presented in his book *I and Thou (Ich und Du, 1923)* for my personal interactions, whether communicating with a person who has dementia or one who is healthy. Buber proposes that human life finds its meaning in relationship, and that relationship is what brings us closer to God. The relationship can be with an animal, a tree, or a rock, as much as it can be between two individuals. Ultimately, the "I" and the "Thou" — I and You — melt into one. When I look into the eyes of another human being I see the reflection of my Self. In upholding Buber's ideal, rather than seeing myself and the person I engage with as separate entities, we would engage in a dialogue involving each other's whole being so that we become a unity of being, without distinct boundaries.

This way of interacting is not easy. It takes time and lots of practice. But while caring for someone with dementia, I found it helpful to remind myself of Buber's philosophy and to try to engage in an I-Thou interaction when I had the energy, patience, and mindfulness.

People living in South Asia are fortunate that they have a way of repeatedly honoring "the other" throughout the day, without being reminded. Hindus, Sikhs, Jains, and Buddhists greet each other and say good-bye to each other by placing their palms together in front of their hearts and saying "namaste." (Thai people say "wie" which is said with a similar gesture.) Variations of the meaning of namaste include: "I greet that place where you and I are one." "The light of God in me recognizes itself in you." "I see and honor in you the place where God resides. When you are at that place in you, and I am at that place in me, we are one."

Of course, it's easy for the greeter to use the salutation as just that, a perfunctory greeting. But the opportunity of recognizing "Thou" as "I" is available numerous times each day to these people.

Creating a beautiful space

A beautiful space nourishes the spirit inside of us. It can stimulate renewal and deep relaxation, so think of ways to enhance your own environment, as well as the room in which the patient spends a lot of time. If you have an extra room in your home, create a sacred space or meditation room where you can retreat and connect with your self. An entire room can invite you into your deeper self. If you don't have an entire room, a corner or closet will do. Here are some helpful ideas:

- Maintain a clean environment without clutter.
- Enjoy a vase of fresh flowers.
- Burn incense to clear and purify the air, unless the smoke or odor is irritating.
- Paint the walls a color that rejuvenates your spirit. For instance, green is healing and relaxing, red restores vitality in people who are depressed, and purple is powerful for those who need spiritual and emotional healing.
- Gather gemstones. They exert healing effects. For instance, lithium quartz is said to ease tension and stress, and keep nightmares at bay. Pink Calcite promotes compassion, healing, and universal love. Amethyst is for protection, purification, and spiritual/divine connection.
- Listening to calming sounds can relax a tense body within minutes. Consider a wind chime, water fountain, or a CD (compact disc) of singing birds, ocean waves, or falling rain.
- Use essential oils or aromatherapy to have a specific effect on the body, mind, and spirit. (See *Aromatherapy*, Chapter 18.)
- Have a supply of pens, markers, and notebooks, in case you want to write in a journal.

- Create an outdoor sacred space with river rocks, a koi or lily pond, a flowering tree or shrub, pampas grass, colored sand — the possibilities are endless.

- Include religious symbols, chakra symbols, animal totems, prayer flags, angel statues, rainbow banners, and lamps with colored bulbs — it's up to you.

- Enjoy the space you are in by remembering to: Stay present. Breathe. Speak sweetly. Be grateful for the good days. Drink water. Eat greens. "Remember that this too shall pass." Note that this is one of the 'mantras' that kept me going.

* * *

References

Carter, Patricia A., Jacquelyn H. Flaskerud, and Patricia Lee. 2009. "Distressing Emotions in Female Caregivers of People with AIDS, Age-Related Dementias, and Advanced-Stage Cancers." *Perspectives in Psychiatric Care*. 36(4):121-3.

Mueller, Paul S., David J. Plevak, and Teresa A. Rummans. 2001. "Religious Involvement, Spirituality, and Medicine: Implications for Clinical Practice." *Mayo Clinic Proceedings*. 76 (12):1225-1235.

Niaura, Raymond, Joan Russo, and Peter P. Vitaliano. 1994. "Plasma Lipids and their Relationships with Psychosocial Factors in Older Adults." *The Journals of Gerontology*. 50B:18-24.

3

The Power of Words

Spoken words have a profound effect on the person they are directed at. Yet, it's not easy to always speak kindly and sweetly when caring for someone who has dementia. This chapter offers ways to be mindful about how we speak to others in trying circumstances, especially the ones we love and cherish.

A word is dead
When it is said, some say.
I say it just begins to live that day.
– Emily Dickinson

On Yom Kippur 2007 (the year 5767 according to the Jewish calendar) Rabbi Marc Soloway of Congregation Bonai Shalom in Boulder, Colorado gave a sermon on the topic of the power of words. Judaism teaches that the power of negative words is the equivalent to murder. In the Talmud to speak *lashon harah* (evil speech or gossip) is like killing three people: the person about whom we are speaking, the person to whom we are talking *and* ourselves.

"We somehow know that however much we regret those words said in anger or in pain, we can never retrieve them. No matter how much we apologize or express regret, the damage has been done and it may be difficult or even impossible to repair," said Rabbi Soloway.

He told a famous story that opens the first chapter of Joseph Telushkin's book *Words that Hurt, Words that Heal*. In an Eastern European village, a man went through the community slandering the rabbi. One day, feeling suddenly remorseful, he begged the rabbi for forgiveness and offered to undergo any penance to make amends. The rabbi told him to take a feather pillow from his home, cut it open, scatter the feathers to the wind, and then return to see him. The man did as he was told, then came to the rabbi and asked, "Am I now forgiven?"

"Almost," came the response. "You just have to do one more thing. Go and gather all the feathers."

"But that's impossible," the man protested. "The wind has already scattered them."

"Precisely," the rabbi answered. "And although you truly wish to correct the evil you have done, it is as impossible to repair the damage done by your words as it is to recover the feathers."

Buddhism similarly teaches that we should be mindful of our actions and especially our speech, and to be acutely aware of the present moment. The Zen monk Thich Nhat Hanh stresses the importance of deep listening and loving speech.

With all this in mind, I try to speak sweetly, mindful of how spoken words can either deeply damage or uplift someone. Alas, this was one of my greatest challenges in caring for someone with Alzheimer's.

Sometimes Morris would say, "Why can't you be nice? Why are you speaking like that?" What he meant was "Why are you cranky? Why can't you speak with compassionate understanding of what I am going through?" He also said, "I don't like you," which always came across sounding like the words uttered by a frustrated, recalcitrant child. But Morris wasn't a child. He was an adult with a terrible disease, and when he said those things, he was absolutely clear in his observation that I was not being nice and that I was unlikable at that moment. After a day — or a morning — of his repeatedly asking me the same question, or my having to explain a simple direction or concept umpteen times, I began to lose it. I did get cranky. I lost my temper and sometimes I shouted at him. It's easy to make excuses, but the reality is that it is not easy to be sweet all the time, or even most of the time, while caregiving day after day.

Take, for instance, the days Morris was particularly resistant against taking his medication and supplements. He hated to take his pills and put up a fight almost every day. We both suffered as a result. And later, when he went to live in the memory care home, his caregivers had the same problem. They came up with all kinds of tactics, including putting his pills in ice cream, which worked for a while. When it got to the point when he was spitting them out, we had to resort to liquid medications that were put in juice.

When Morris was living at home, on days that he felt sick to his stomach I only gave him the essential drugs. He usually took herbs to uplift his spirit and reduce anxiety. When the herbs were omitted from the daily regimen, it became very apparent. Morris got moodier, more defiant, and harder to be around. And that made things more difficult for me. On more than one occasion I witnessed hot anger pour out of my mouth, "Take your fucking pills!" I shocked myself. I can count on one hand the number of times I had ever used the "F word."

Morris was as shocked as I was when I shouted at him. His head would drop and he'd frown. He'd sit at the table folding into himself like a scolded child, and after a five-minute sulk, would finally take his pills without further argument. This would lead to our exchanging apologies and a serious discussion about where the Alzheimer's came from. I told him that scientists still do not know, and when they make that discovery they will also find a cure. Morris would then tell me how he was doing the best that he could.

In Morris's words — March 2007

One time I feel one way and another time I feel a different way. I cope by finding things to do. I read, talk to people, go out to lunch with my friends. I feel just like anybody else, but I'm limited in things that I want to do, or where I want to go. I have to have someone take care of me. I would rather be my own person and do what I can do as much as possible. It's not great having this [Alzheimer's] and there's not much I can do about it. But I do have lots of great friends and family, and I'm lucky to be able to think and act and live a partial life.

I'm not very happy at times. It's not easy for me, and my wife tries to help as much as possible. I feel frustrated. I can't have my car, which was taken away. I don't have as many options. We have our TM lunch*; one of the things I look forward to. That's a happy thing to do. Having people around is obviously good. I like watching movies and TV.

Sometimes I don't know what to do, or I forget things and have to depend on my wife. I've had things taken away from me. When I first got the diagnosis, I thought it was a bunch of crap. I didn't think the doctor had the right diagnosis and that I was pretty much okay. Now I understand that I have Alzheimer's disease and things are more difficult. That's the way it is. Having a support group is very important to me. Sometimes I get frustrated and sometimes I feel that I'm still a human being and that I can do things.

I know I'm taken care of. I'm able to just be a good person that other people want to be around. I'm already enlightened in my own way. I feel like I'm my own being, my own person, and am living a life to the best of my ability. I like music and culture. I'm very lucky to have a support group of friends and family. In this life, I'm doing the best I can and I'll continue to with friends and family.

I want to be treated like any other human being. My message to others is try to find your own happiness and do the best you can. I still like to meditate and I like to take a nap every day. I am getting more tired. I can't do a lot or do as well as I used to do.

About a dozen friends who practice Transcendental Meditation have been meeting regularly for lunch every Tuesday for the past 18 years.

* * *

So how does speaking hurtfully fit in with my paradigm of operating in the world as a loving, compassionate person who strives to be mindful about what I do? It doesn't. I was, and am continually striving to be, more patient and compassionate, which developed into a spiritual quest. Transcendental Meditation, the mantra-based meditation that I practice, certainly helps. The instruction is to come back to the mantra when the mind realizes it is thinking thoughts. It's done gently without force or strain, and after the meditation practice, I emerge rested, clear, and alert so that I can continue with my day.

When Morris alerted me that I was being bitchy, I stepped back, took a breath, and went back to my *center*. It's meditation in action. I take a deep breath, see the situation from the other person's perspective, and pull in the reins. With Morris, I apologized and stepped outside of myself for a moment to take a closer look at his needs and why I was acting the way I was. Then I stepped back inside myself with a better understanding of what I needed to do in order to re-establish harmony. It sounds too simple, but it does work — it did work — *when* I was capable of doing it. Sometimes, if either Morris or I was having a particularly rough day, I had to leave the house to regain my composure and sense of control over my emotions, and to simply recharge my batteries. When I returned, I was able to again speak gently. I forgave myself and forgave Morris.

It helped me to remember this saying from Vedic literature: "satyam bruyat, priyam bruyat," which means *speak the sweet truth*. Speaking sweetly helps create joy and health in the body. Speaking angrily creates fire, irritation, and inflammation. It makes us feel bad, and hurts the person who hears our angry words. Practicing unconditional forgiveness helps to quash the seed of anger before it turns into an inferno.

4

Living in the Now

It's hard not to focus on the future when you and a family member receive a devastating medical prognosis. In fact, the future might be the first thing you frantically consider; it might overwhelm your thoughts entirely. Here are some techniques, rituals, and affirmations to help you maintain a positive outlook throughout the day and enjoy the time you have with your care partner, here and now.

> "Live quietly in the moment and see the beauty of all before you. The future will take care of itself..."
> – Paramahansa Yogananda, *Autobiography of a Yogi*

After Morris was diagnosed, I cried for a solid month. I'd wake up every hour or so during the night, crying and worrying about the future. Although I never had a full-blown panic attack, I was in a continual state of panic, thinking, "What happens when Morris is unable to recognize us? What happens when he can no longer drive? Will I have to put him in a nursing home? Will I have enough money?"

The questions would grip my mind and squeeze tears onto my pillow until I fell into an exhausted sleep. The cycle would repeat itself all night long. The same fearful thoughts intruded my day, only to be shoved into the background when I managed to write or tend to household chores. I discovered Eckhart Tolle's book *The Power of Now: A Guide to Spiritual Enlightenment,* which is what I credit with saving my sanity. It helped me learn how to stay focused on the present—the here and now.

When you realize that the present is the only thing that is real, it frees you from the fear of what is to come. Even though you might have an idea of what the future holds, from a medical prognosis or an astrology reading, if you stay focused on the present, you can avoid the emotions that get triggered when you think about putting someone in a nursing home…or running out of money… or losing a spouse. The list goes on and on.

The reality of life is that we don't know what will happen tomorrow. The only reality is what is happening right now in this moment. When you find yourself getting scared and fearful about what might happen tomorrow or next week or in a year from now, stop and ask yourself this, "How do I feel right now, this second?" Most of the time you'll answer, "Okay. I'm okay right now." You might not be okay in an hour from now, or tomorrow, but you can loosen the grip of fear when you come back to the absolute present, which is NOW. Of course, in dealing with practicalities, we have to plan for the future. Writing a will, filling out medical directives, making a doctor's appointment, and taking the car in to get serviced require us to think about the future.

It's easy — and natural — to become preoccupied with future events. Ancient Vedic texts describe the human mind as a monkey jumping from branch to branch, until it is trained to settle down and experience pure consciousness, or the source from where all thoughts originate. People have a tendency to play different scenarios over and over in their minds about what can happen if we make a certain decision or act in a particular way. Most of the time those scenarios are seldom realized. We play them out in our minds and they fade away after causing us to lose sleep and wreaking havoc on our emotions and overall health.

Training my mind to stay in the present was one of the greatest tools that helped me to get through the day, the weeks, the months, and the years of caring for someone with a chronic, terminal disease. During the day when I found myself thinking about a future event or outcome such as, *"what will we do when we run out of money?"* I reminded myself to come back to the here and now, and that my thoughts about the past or future were not part of my reality. This technique definitely helped to dispel my worries about the future and helped me maintain peace of mind, which helped me stay calmer and more patient with Morris. And although it sounds contradictory, staying emotionally and mentally grounded in the present helped me maintain the mental clarity necessary for making future arrangements. Staying present is a valuable technique that I incorporated into my spiritual practice then, and which I still use and will continue to use.

A ritual to help you and your care partner enjoy the "here and now"

Learning how to stay present enhances how you relate to the person you are caring for, allowing you to create community with that person. The simple act of breathing with someone—of matching your breath to his or hers—enables you to create a spiritual connection with that person.

Light a candle to create a soothing space. Place two chairs side by side or facing one another.

Ask your care partner to sit comfortably.

Just breathe in and out, matching his or her breath.

Hold the person's hand, if you like, and speak sweetly or sing together, staying in the present moment. Read a poem, chant or pray together, or listen to music. Enjoy the moment. It will never repeat itself in exactly the same way.

10 Affirmations to set the tone of the day

Before you get out of bed in the morning, breathe deeply through your nose several times. Scan your body for any aches or pains. Feel them and be with them for a moment, and then imagine a golden light piercing them like a sword. Next, choose one of the following affirmations to repeat silently or quietly for a minute or two.

1. I'm feeling strong and healthy today.
2. I will make the right decisions today for my care partner and myself.
3. I feel love for all living things.
4. I am a kind, compassionate caregiver.
5. I am grateful for the love that surrounds me.

6. I will remain calm and patient throughout the day.

7. Today I will do the best that I can.

8. I welcome peace, trust, and acceptance into my life.

9. Today I will let things unfold without worrying about every consequence.

10. Today I will speak sweetly with kindness and patience.

5

The Comfort of Rituals

Everyone grieves in different ways. This chapter provides an understanding of the losses that accompany anticipatory grief, universal rituals that help us to let go with greater compassion and understanding, and a beautiful ritual for saying good-bye to someone who has become a "ghost" of their former self.

"Your sacred space is where you can find yourself
over and over again."
– Joseph Campbell

Since Alzheimer's disease is a fatal disease, families of Alzheimer's patients experience anticipatory grief sometimes for years before the patient actually dies. The ill patient also experiences grief when the car keys are taken away, or when he or she can't read any longer or participate in a favorite activity. According to clinical psychologist Therese Rando, PhD, who expanded the initial concept of anticipatory grief, there are three types of losses that occur as part of anticipated grief.

- Past losses in terms of lost opportunities and past experiences that will not be repeated
- Present losses in terms of the progressive deterioration of the ill person, and the uncertainty and loss of control
- Future losses that will occur as a consequence of the loved one's illness and eventual death, including economic uncertainty, loneliness, a change in lifestyle, and even loss of purpose when the caregiving ends

Public rituals such as funerals and memorial services are performed after a person dies. But you don't have to wait until after a loved one passes to create a ritual to help you gain control and face your grief while your loved one slips further into the disease. Writing letters, journaling (see *Journaling*, Chapter 27), having imaginary conversations with your loved one, listening to the music you both loved, walking in the woods, or even just perusing photo albums and remembering the happy times you shared can help you feel more in control and in touch with your feelings.

Here's a very beautiful and powerful ritual for saying good-bye to a memory-impaired loved one while that person is still alive.

Lamenting Our Losses: Rituals for Coping with Dementia

By **Linda Loewenstein** and **David J. Zucker**

Learning about the death of someone is always shocking, although it may or may not be surprising. Death is just so ... final. It is indisputably the end of that living relationship. Nevertheless, even in its finality, there is something certain, something definable. Further, our society has certain rituals that surround death. The laws of each state define burial practices. Each religious tradition addresses mourning practices. There are boundaries, accepted norms of behavior, even pre-printed notes that thank our friends for their heartfelt condolences. All of these defined expectations provide a framework as people struggle through feelings of loss and despair. The defined rituals buttress the mourners as they continue to live in the lonely fog that follows the death of a loved one.

But, there are those of us who have a relative lost in the ravages of dementia. The person we knew and loved is gone, yet a shadow of that person exists. How can we mourn the loss while simultaneously respecting the living being that contains the remnants of the person we loved?

Caring for a loved one with dementia is a daunting prospect. Without rituals, without the overt acknowledgement that a monumental change has occurred, we struggle in a spiritual wilderness. Relatives and friends do not have any kind of ritualized way to acknowledge their *ongoing* sense of diminishment and grief at the fact that they no longer have that person in their lives in any kind of meaningful or communicable way.

Rituals can highlight changes in our lives. Some Jewish rituals reflect changes in time or space—for example, the ritual welcoming Shabbat on Friday night, the ritual blessing you say when you move into a new home, the joyous "*Shehehiyanu*," a blessing said when there is something unique, or reaching a significant milestone in life. The ritualization serves as our acknowledgement, both internal and external, of something new, special, or different.

Lamenting our losses: the rituals

The rituals that we list below are designed for the person who feels the sense of loss. They may be performed alone or you may choose to include others—family or close friends who are aware of your losses. Although it might be possible to include the loved one whose diminishment you're lamenting, it may be easier initially to experience the ritual without that added layer. Obviously, this is a personal experience, and a matter of personal choice. The frequency of the ritual(s) is also an individual matter. You may find that this helps on a weekly basis, or it might be monthly or quarterly. You may be completely arbitrary in terms of its frequency; a stand alone, once-only event, or it might be a ritual you repeat with long spaces of time in between.

The Five Stages

1. Preparation
2. Candle Ceremony
3. Living Eulogy
4. Prayers and Pleas
5. Conclusion/Closure

Preparation

Items:

Two large candles (Shabbat candles are fine), a knife, matches

Three candleholders

In a safe and comforting space, you will cut one of the candles. Literally cutting the candle is symbolic. In the physical act of cutting, you acknowledge that there has been a break, a significant rupture with the past. By cutting the thread/wick within the candle, you affirm that what had been the thread of connection has been irretrievably and irreparably severed. Perhaps your loved one no longer recognizes you, or the person is no longer able to interact with their environment, or no longer able to maintain a friendship from the past. In addition, the act of cutting echoes, but does not literally replicate, the Jewish ritual of *Keriyah* (literally "cutting/rending" — the tradition of placing a cut in one's garment as a sign of mourning, based on biblical verses in Genesis 37:34 and Job 1:20). Mourners who are in one of the following relationships perform the ritual of *Keriyah* — for one's father, mother, sister, brother, wife, husband, son, or daughter.

Recite these words just before you cut the candle:

Ba-rukh atta Ado-nai, Elo-hey-nu mekor ḥayim, al d'var k'ritut.

Praised are You, Eternal our God, source of life, concerning the matter of "cutting."

Take the candle and cut it unevenly, approximately 2/3 and 1/3. You will then have three candles — one full length and two others of differing shorter lengths. The three candles represent three different periods of time — the past, the present, and the future. The longest candle symbolizes the past — the part of memory that is the largest, the time period that is most likely to remain accessible to a person experiencing dementia. It is the most solid and least likely to completely disappear. The present — the middle-sized candle — is less full and more tenuous. The smallest candle represents the future — a short period of time, either real time or the time left for meaningful interaction.

Candle Ceremony

"Acknowledging the Diminishing Light"

Place the three candles in candleholders and light them. You can choose to say one of the following blessings. These blessings, which focus on light and life/living, are reminiscent of the Saturday night *Havdalah* ritual that marks the division (*havdalah*) between Shabbat (Sabbath) and the normal weekdays. This entire "Lamenting our Losses" ceremony/ritual highlights the division between the life that was and the life that is now.

Recite one of the following prayers; the one that best expresses how you feel about the stages of your loved one's journey.

> *Ba-rukh atta Ado-nai, Elo-hey-nu mekor ḥayim, borey or,*
> *u-mav-dil beyn heh-ḥayim, v' heh-ḥai.*

Praised are You, Eternal our God, source of life, who creates Light, and distinguishes between Living and Life

(or)

> *Ba-rukh atta Ado-nai, Elo-hey-nu mekor ḥayim, borcy or,*
> *u-mav-dil beyn heh-ḥai, v' heh-ḥayim.*

Praised are You, Eternal our God, source of life, who creates Light, and distinguishes between Life and Living

(or)

> *Ba-rukh atta Ado-nai, Elo-hey-nu mekor ḥayim, borey or,*
> *u-mav-dil beyn ḥayim, l'ḥayim.*

Praised are You, Eternal our God, source of life, who creates Light, and distinguishes between Living and Living.

Meditation

At this time, as I light these candles, I seek the inner strength and courage to help me light the way to work through the pain of the sense of loss and abandonment that I feel within. I grieve the relationships that were so important to me in past days, and I seek enlightenment and insight so that I will achieve healing within myself and be of comfort to the one I love.

Living Eulogy

The Living Eulogy, similar to a eulogy delivered at a funeral, is an acknowledgment and tribute to the person who was/is so important in your life. A funeral eulogy can serve as an instrument of closure. In the case of this Living Eulogy, closure in the sense of a "final closure" is not possible; the person is still living, although he/she is not accessible (or not fully accessible) because of the dementia. The Living Eulogy is something that you, yourself, write. It may be a paragraph, a page, or several pages long. It may be just a memory of a single event. It recalls parts of the life of the person who is there, but curiously, not there. Instead of, or in addition to, something written, you may also choose to find a favorite photograph of your loved one, a photograph that reminds you of the person's wholeness. Some of the people who might be present at this ceremony may want to add their own words, either extemporaneously, or through words prepared beforehand.

We suggest that you save the words of the Living Eulogy after the ceremony. At a later date, it might be the basis for another Living Eulogy that you write for the next time(s) you perform this ritual. And when, eventually, the person dies, these Living Eulogies can form part of the funeral eulogy.

Prayers and Pleas

This next section, Prayers and Pleas, are longer expressions of the grief and ongoing grieving and loss that you are experiencing. We have offered several examples or suggestions. You might choose to use these models or create your own prayers and pleas.

A prayer about memory

Ba-rukh atta Ado-nai, Elo-hey-nu me-lekh ha-olam, a-sher m'kadesh et amo al y'dei zikhronot.

Praised are You, Eternal our God, ruler of the world, who makes people holy through memory.

(or)

Source of goodness and blessing, strength and holiness, may this be a sacred moment devoted to memory.

Embracing their truth

Help me understand that there is a difference between what is "true" (for my loved one) and what are the actual facts. May I learn to embrace and affirm their truth, irrespective of actual or demonstrable facts.

Allow me to hear words that pain me, words that shame me, without armoring myself with defensive weapons. Help me to understand that fear has tampered with reality.

A prayer for the person I have lost

I will be with you in your difficult journey ahead, sometimes physically with you, sometimes spiritually. I will be there, even when you feel, think, or say that I am not.

Self-care

Let me not look for signposts where there are none, interpret meaning when there is none, hope when there is no chance. Allow me to accept, to be, instead of to do.

As we journey through this vast desert, help me to create an emotional oasis, a place where I can rest and renew.

How can I know?

- How do I know where you are when I cannot read the signposts?
- How do I find you in the dense forest that shelters you?
- How can I reach you when my arms are not long enough?

- How can I know if you are at peace? Is your silence from paralyzing fear or a response to God's comforting embrace?
- Do you see flashes of reds and orange, or is your world gray?
- Do you understand any of my words; find any comfort in the cadence of my voice?
- How can I know if you are at peace?
- I must believe; believe in a God of mercy, and believe in God's grace.

A silent confession

- I have failed to understand that the physical items surrounding you, the accumulation and debris of ordinary life, provide you comfort as your mental cupboard becomes increasingly bare.
- I have failed fully to comprehend that your continually asked question is new to you each time it is voiced.
- I have failed to understand that as much as I hate your life, you hate it even more.
- I have run from your presence, gladly distancing myself while asking others to endure the unendurable. Remind me to honor those whose patience is greater than mine.
- I have repeatedly attempted to use logic and reason while knowing that the more effective tools are affirmation and diversion. Help me to remember that your seemingly ordinary language masks your confusion and that words are not always an appropriate tool.
- I have maintained a pace that suits me, forgetting that the speeding train of life must slow at dementia's crossroads.
- I have cursed the medications that you take that prolong my agony of watching you deteriorate. Please help me treasure those disappearing remnants of your being that still speak of your wholeness.

- I have used the private tragedy of your current existence as conversational currency. Please allow others to understand that my pain is often soothed by the balm of social support.

- Please help me to provide moments of joy and happiness amid your fear and loneliness.

Conclusion/Closure

At this point, the ritual is over and before blowing out the candles, you may choose to conclude in any way that feels appropriate.

In Jewish tradition, the prophet Elijah never died, but was taken into heaven on a fiery chariot. He continues to live, and is understood to be ever present, ready to help in moments of danger or distress. Elijah also is credited with revealing hidden truths. He is a celestial connection, and is featured in the closing words of the prophet Malachi, where Malachi speaks of Elijah "reconciling parents with children and children with their parents" (Malachi 3:24 Hebrew; alternatively Malachi 4:5). Coincidentally, at the close of the *Havdalah* ceremony, which marks divisions in time, it is traditional to sing of Elijah. Consequently, one way you may choose to conclude this ritual is to sing softly the words of that hymn:

Eli-ya-hu ha na-vi, Eli-ya-hu ha-Tish-bi, Eli-ya-hu, Eli-ya-hu, Eli-ya-hu ha-Gi-la-di.

Bim-hey-ra b'ya-mey-nu, Ya-vo a-ley-nu, im ma-shi-ah ben-David, im ma-shi-ah ben David.

Elijah the prophet, Elijah the [person from] Tishbi, Elijah the [person from] Gil'ad.

Quickly in our time, come to us, with the Messiah, the son of David.

(At the close of this ritual, you will blow out the candles. You can use them again. In time, the smallest candle will burn out and the other candles will be shortened. If/when this ritual is repeated, use a new large candle.)

* * *

Authors Loewenstein and Zucker are Jewish professionals in the Met-ro-Denver area, and they collaborated on the ritual described above. Loewenstein's perspective is that of a family member, as she describes, "My mother is suffering from Alzheimer's disease. It's a brutal process and I have felt spiritually adrift. I find myself talking about her as if she was dead, yet she's not dead. This new damaged being is not my mother, even though there are flashes of my mother. This version of my mother seems like a badly handicapped twin sister – not really my mother at all. For the past couple of years, I have needed some way to identify and acknowledge this shift in my universe. I have yearned for a comforting ritual to help me walk this long and difficult path."

Zucker is a rabbi and full-time chaplain at Shalom Park, a senior contin-uum of care center in Denver, Colorado. In that latter capacity, he created the Resident's Family Support Group, designed to meet the ongoing needs of families around issues of loss, frustration, anger, helplessness, and grief. "In counseling with families," explains Rabbi Zucker, "I began to understand that there are common threads in their stories. Children, spouses, significant others, and siblings need time and a safe place to vent, to lament, and to share a commonality of mutual sorrow." Find more information by visiting his website, <u>www.davidjzucker.org</u>.

6

Caregiver Guilt and Compassion

Caregivers can often feel guilty when taking care of a terminally ill family member. Am I doing enough? Did I make the right decision? What if... what if...? Here are ways to recognize your feelings, tips for accepting them, and ways to forgive yourself.

"Even when muddy, your wings sparkle bright wonders that heal broken worlds."
– Aberjhani, *The River of Winged Dreams*

Some philosophers and psychologists believe guilt is mental and emotional anguish that is culturally imposed on us. Tibetans and Native Americans don't even have a word for guilt, which might mean that it isn't a basic human emotion. Yet, Jews and Christians are very adept at feeling guilty over trivial mistakes, as well as serious blunders.

The first time I felt guilt was when my brother was born. I'm two years older than he, and in 1954 the hospital rules didn't allow siblings to visit newborns. My Uncle Irv placed me on his shoulders so I could see my mother, who waved to me from the window of her hospital room. I was angry with her for leaving me and I refused to look at her. She waved like the beautiful lady in the fancy red car that passed me by in the Memorial Day parade. But I wouldn't look at her. The memory is a black and white movie that has replayed itself throughout my life, with the film always breaking at the point when I sullenly turn my head away.

For years afterwards, I would awaken in the night feeling guilty that I didn't look at her. When I was four years old, I fell out of bed onto the wooden floor of the bedroom I shared with my brother because I was having a bad dream. I don't recall the dream, but I remember the ache inside my chest that has always been associated with not doing what my mother wanted me, or expected me, to do.

Over the years, up until my early fifties, I'd have a physical sensation that felt like sand paper or grains of sand inside the skin of my hands that would migrate to the skin and muscles of my arms and torso. Sometimes it felt like my arms and hands were paralyzed or had grown in size. It was hard to move, and the uneasiness of guilt was always associated with the sensation. I recently realized that I haven't felt those sensations in a very long time.

Maybe I lost those sensations because the guilt of my childhood was replaced by the guilt I felt over placing Morris in a memory care home. I could have taken care of him until the end of his life, but I was drowning in misery and I promised myself I wouldn't sacrifice everything for this illness. I prayed for his release and my relief, and knew that if I had taken care of him until the end, my own health would have suffered.

I tried to help Morris fight Alzheimer's by bringing him to healers, holy people, and complementary medicine practitioners. I fed him an organic, whole-foods diet and gave him nutritional supplements, in addition to the prescribed pharmaceutical drugs. I ordered a drug from Europe before it was FDA approved and prescribed as part of the Alzheimer's drug protocol by U.S. physicians. I did all this until I finally realized that Morris needed to take the solitary journey of being a victim of Alzheimer's disease. Some call it fate and others call it karma. Whatever we name it, no matter how much we are loved and in close communion with family and friends, we have to travel the delicate path of life on our own. When we succumb to illness and disease, it becomes especially painful for others to helplessly stand by and watch, after doing everything humanly possible to assist.

There was always one more "magic bullet" for Morris to try, and yet, when I felt the possibility of divine intervention weaken, I began to give up hope and let destiny take its course. The first couple of years after Morris's passing, the guilt—and grief—would unexpectedly grab me, wrapping its tentacles around my chest. It would twist the insides of my stomach, making it impossible to eat. It would swell into a lump in my throat or tighten a band around my head, destroying my serenity for an hour or two —or an entire day.

Guilt came in layers, piled up like the blankets I tossed from my bed one by one during a cold winter's night. The blankets came off as my temperature rose and drops of sweat pooled between my breasts. I shook off the feelings of guilt in a similar way when I heard my therapist's words in the back of my mind reminding me that I did more than I could do; when I remembered that I'm a mere mortal who breaks and cries when I can't move one more inch beyond the confines of this physical body; when my heart had expanded to the point where it can't expand anymore, so it has to contract in order to plow through the walls of pain and deal with the guilt.

Why do I still feel guilt? I feel guilt about not being the perfect wife before Morris got sick. This man adored me and I didn't reciprocate with a passion that matched his. I feel guilt because I'm alive and he's not. (Survivor's guilt is commonly felt by those who share in a tragic event in which the cherished partner dies, leaving the other one to live and put back the pieces of the life they once shared.) I feel guilt about the times I could have spent with Morris watching television or taking a walk instead of running out to be with friends or to dance. Feeling guilt for doing anything to get away from his asking me the same question over and over again, or so I wouldn't have to watch the man who once stood tall and proud, stoop and stumble like a man way beyond his years.

I hear the therapist's voice in my head asking, "What would you say to someone who just told you all this?"

I'd say, "But you did the absolute best that you could do." And then I feel better. It's okay. I'm okay. I really did the best I knew how, and Morris lived longer than his prognosis because of it. Now, several years after his passing, the guilt appears much less frequently. It hovers momentarily like a hummingbird poking its beak into honeysuckle and hollyhock. The guilt is diluted and flavorless like cream that's been frozen without added fruit or chocolate chips. It's a color without pigment, a touch without pressure, a sound without notes. The guilt I feel now is background noise; not noticed until I turn off the other sounds in my world or mindlessly drive my car on a dark, damp day, which is unusual in sunny Colorado. The guilt now appears in various shades of dirty white and brown. It doesn't reach inside my heart with its claw like it used to. The battle is over, but not completely finished.

Tips for easing guilt

Ask yourself what is bothering you. Talk with a close friend who will not judge you, or with a professional therapist, clergy person, spiritual teacher, or intuitive guide. Talk about your guilt until you feel your body release the tension that is stored in your muscles and cells.

Remember that you are human and not perfect. No one expects you to perform with absolute clarity and grace all the time.

You cannot control everything all the time. You are doing the best that you can with the information, strength, and inner resources that you have.

Have an "empty chair" dialogue by speaking out loud and pretending that your care partner is in the chair next to you. Express your feelings openly and wholeheartedly. Ask for forgiveness if you feel that you wronged your loved one in any way.

Write down your thoughts and feelings. (See Journaling, Chapter 27)

Strong feelings of guilt, remorse, and grief will diminish over time. If they continue to haunt you, seek professional help.

Part Two

X

Caregivers' Stories

7

Finding Love and Forgiveness as Patient and Caregiver

By **Adele Britton**

I had rock-solid trust in Paul, the wonderful man I had married in 1985, to remain identifiable as "Paul" for the duration of our lives together. I had absolute faith and trust in him. I don't know if I've ever felt that way about anyone else. I was so positive that we had everything covered to 'do it right.' We had read all the right books, taken good care of ourselves, exercised, discussed everything deeply, and enjoyed good health. We were good lovers and friends, and walked hand in hand through life's ups and downs. When we had a problem, we discussed it and taught others how to cope with life's challenges — both as professionals and role models. We were also very independent within our marriage. Paul and I did our own things, and when we came together, it was to share. As far as we were concerned, we had it made.

But my husband's ability to think straight, to reason adroitly, and especially to remember names, places, and things began to collapse thirteen years after we married, when he was sixty-two years old. A lot of times I'd miss it, since he was so brilliant and was able to compensate for his lapses. I noticed that he had to write things down in order to remember them. Now, all these years later, it's apparent that when we held hands crossing the street and it seemed as though he was guiding me or hustling me and I'd say, annoyed, "I'm not a child," he didn't want to hold my hand because he was being affectionate. He was holding my hand because, when we crossed the street, he became rigid and startled by the traffic noise. He was frightened. Sounds like car doors and the garage door being closed would also startle him. But I thought his oversensitivity and forgetfulness was from stress.

Paul was always very social and did well in groups. When we went to Costa Rica in 1997, I noticed that he didn't want to join in the group activities as much and was quite reticent. When he was climbing up into the rainforest canopy, the group on the ground called him "Papa Grande" because he was presenting himself as an old man.

Paul recognized there was something wrong. We went to our family physician, who sent us to a memory center for testing. It was all there in black and white. Paul did poorly on the Mini-Mental State Examination (MMSE), and an MRI showed brain shrinkage. The MMSE is a brief thirty point questionnaire used to assess cognition. It includes simple questions and problems in a number of areas: the time and place of the test, repeating lists of words, arithmetic, language use and comprehension, and copying a drawing. At that point, it was suggested that Paul see a neurologist. It took a while for him to agree; because even in his compromised state, Paul was more aware and available mentally and emotionally than the average person. When the neurologist told him to surrender his car keys, Paul was very angry and said, "I haven't had an accident yet."

Perhaps it was then, during the dawning of the horrifying grief and responsibility I knew I'd be facing, that my own devastating infirmity began developing in my body. By 2003, when Paul was actually diagnosed with Alzheimer's at the age sixty-seven, I was stressed and weary, and unaware that a year later I would join the ranks of the 50-60% of caregiving spouses who are stricken with an autoimmune disease. I was working desperately hard, trying to take care of Paul and keep our lives afloat and manageable, when I learned that I had contracted a rare, incurable, and potentially fatal blood disease called amyloidosis. Struggling for my life, I underwent months of chemotherapy and then had a bone marrow transplant. Paul and I were, indeed, a sorry tangle of illness, upheaval, and enormous uncertainty.

Yet instead of suffering, I chose to transcend my problems and focus on healing my mind. I knew that my thoughts about my situation would influence how I would react to everything that was happening. I became a keen observer and a decider. I stopped taking everything so seriously; in fact, I started to see humor, irony, and absurdity everywhere. When I considered the question, "What if the hokey pokey is what it's all about?" To my great delight, it struck me that everything that is not love is hokey pokey. I decided to turn my challenging state of affairs into something profoundly valuable by accepting love into my life and refusing anything else.

For the past thirty-four years I've been a student of A Course in Miracles (also referred to as ACIM or the Course, it is a book containing a self-study curriculum of spiritual transformation written by Helen Schucman from 1965 to 1972). My spiritual path has led me to believe that what we call life is really an elaborate dream, an illusion in which everything that happens is purposeful, even perfect. And further, that I am not a victim of my circumstances but have, in fact, called these events into my life as a precise way to learn about love and forgiveness. I believe that when I respond from pure forgiveness, I am invoking my Highest Self, the place within me that is at peace and union with God. I am imbued with clarity.

Mostly, I have been able to step back from both Paul's and my illness and think about my attitudes, feelings, decisions, and judgments. Not wanting to live my life by default, but by choice, I have asked and answered questions such as "Am I choosing to look at this through the eyes of love or fear? Am I remembering that this 'problem' is a self-chosen lesson in forgiveness?" When I ask myself, "What is this (pain, challenge, sickness, loss) for?" Always, the answer is to remember myself and my husband (as well as others) as only Love.

By not identifying with my body, my illness, or my caregiving responsibilities, I've remained largely lighthearted and at peace. It has also been essential to my healing and well-being, to forgive myself for being sick — and also to forgive Paul for his Alzheimer's. I've had to become diligently self-aware to uncover and forgive the deeply hidden guilt, anger, and resentment that I have felt about the turn our lives have taken, and release us both from our mistakes and missteps along the way.

Earlier, I had lots of anger and hurt, and I felt betrayed that he had abandoned me. I projected that anger at Paul, feeling that he was taking something away from me and was doing something horrible to me. I had unconscious guilt about it, and I was hurting myself by blaming him with my thoughts.

Now I can honestly say from the bottom of my heart that today I have no anger. Paul is on a vital journey of his own making, as am I. I don't condemn his Alzheimer's or resist it. Death of a body is not the end. Seeing the sick as diminished is to see them — and ourselves — fearfully. To perceive someone who is ill as eternal Love, Light, and Spirit is the way we bless and honor them — and ourselves. My husband's disease, along with my own, has provided me with a most lofty purpose. It has been a powerful reminder that we can never be separated from Love.

I'm finally ready to start clearing out stuff. I've gotten rid of boxes of books about healing and am understanding why this was such a shocking thing. We had done everything we could have done to mitigate this. I was bemused. How ridiculous it is to think that there's something to be done when this is our destiny.

When I brought Paul to the nursing home, I said to him, "Will you ever forgive me?" He answered, "Go and be happy." He has released me so he can just be. He doesn't want to be messed with anymore.

Nowadays, he sees an imaginary person and dog and talks to them. They are his friends. I'm not important at all. He hasn't known my name for about a year. When I asked him to identify family members he pointed to me and said, "mother." He pointed to our daughter and said, "daughter." Now he just knows that I'm familiar. He responds to affection, love, and hugs. There are even times when I look at him and think, "Paul, isn't this silly, ridiculous?" I'll start laughing and then he starts laughing. But it's not about him. It's about how I perceive the situation. What we had was a chapter, an era; and for me to hold onto that just keeps us both in bondage.

I'm using this time to remember myself as myself, to be with myself joyfully, and to celebrate my independence. I'm open to things, doing things. To this day, I have no idea about what I'll do in the future. I have no sense of it at all. I'm healthy now and I feel good. I have lots of enthusiasm and curiosity, but mostly acceptance. It will be interesting to see what classes my higher self takes in the schoolroom of life.

Adele's husband Paul peacefully passed away
on October 19, 2007.

* * *

Adele Britton Meffley *was a counselor and co-author with Jenny Atch-ley of* The Hokey Pokey IS What It's All About: Words of Wisdom for the Stressed, the Overworked, the Diagnosed, and Those Who Love Them. *Her work was based primarily on* A Course in Miracles. *She lived in Boulder, Colorado, remarried in 2008, and passed away on September 19, 2012 at age sixty-five from complications due to amyloidosis.*

Chapter 8

The Long Distance Caregiver

By **Julie Carpenter**, MD

My dad lived in Schenectady, New York where he was initially a professor and later professor emeritus at Union College. He taught statistics and trained PhD candidates. According to his students, he was a savant with a calculator in his head, like the character in the movie *Rain Man*. Dad had a genius mind, but he couldn't fix a toilet and he didn't have many social skills. He learned his social skills from my mom, who fixed everything, and they had a fulfilling marriage of over fifty-three years.

The first indication that there was something wrong with Dad, age eighty, was not a typical memory issue. We noticed that when he was in a crowd, he'd suddenly get agitated and so upset that we would have to leave. In 1988, when my son Toby was graduating from sixth grade, I took him on a trip to Washington D.C. with my parents. We went to a fair on the banks of the Potomac River and Dad freaked out in the crowd. It was too stressful for him, and we had to get out of there. That started happening when my parents went to church. It was very embarrassing for my mom.

My parents loved to travel and the last trip my parents took was to Casablanca, Morocco in 1989 to see my sister. Dad was always a great walker and he typically took a long walk every day. In Morocco, he went for a walk and couldn't find his way back to the place where they were staying. After several hours in a restaurant visiting with people there (he was very personable), he finally realized he could call the embassy where my sister worked to let someone know where he was. Meanwhile, my mom and sister were crazy with worry. After that incident, he never again went on a trip away from home.

Dad lost his spatial orientation earlier than he lost his short-term memory. A couple of years before he died, we were all driving home from a movie. He entered the freeway via the off ramp. Luckily we noticed, and that was the end of his driving at night.

A few months later, my mom was in the front yard picking weeds and Dad drove the car over her leg. Fortunately, her leg did not break. That was the end of his driving the car.

Dad gradually became more socially isolated. But he continued to walk and we'd go on walks together. He would stop and smell the roses and comment about everything. He walked up until the last six months of his life, when he started getting lost in the neighborhood and didn't want to go out anymore.

My mom was an exceptional caregiver. I talked to her all the time on the phone, but I mainly helped with practical details and by giving her emotional support. I didn't do any hands-on caregiving, except when I went back to take care of Dad when she was in the hospital. I didn't hold a candle to her, as far as caregiving goes. When I couldn't get Dad to eat or drink, he'd say, "Where is the other one?"

I saw them a couple of times a year. They lived simply and were financially independent. We all had Christmas at their home a year before Dad died. Although he couldn't take care of stocks or financial stuff by the time he was five years into the disease process, that Christmas he still knew who I was and who my kids were.

Mom took care of Dad until the end. The last two months, though she was reluctant, I convinced her to bring in hospice care so she could have some relief. Dad was on a blood thinner at the end and had a pacemaker. He was already pretty far into the Alzheimer's when he got the pacemaker and declined a lot after that. It was hard from my point of view as a doctor, and I'm not sure if his getting the pacemaker was something they should have done. But he never took any drugs for Alzheimer's disease.

Dad was independent until near the end. He was still getting up and getting dressed and he could go to the bathroom by himself. He'd sit at the table and pretend to read the newspaper. But he wouldn't have eaten if my mom or someone hadn't made food for him. One day I was taking care of him and he called his stockbroker and was babbling. There was enough in his brain that he wanted to say, but he couldn't make it come out. He couldn't even speak. Those are the sorts of things that I felt a lot of compassion for; not just because he was my dad, but for anyone with dementia.

Dad's mother and his two sisters also had Alzheimer's disease, and he lived longer than any of them. Even though there is a strong family history, I don't worry about myself getting the disease. I feel that my soul is on a journey, and whatever comes is part of that. Dying from Alzheimer's is not the worst way to go. And if one remains happy, it's not so bad for the family. As a physician, I see people die in excruciating pain. It is a blessing that most people with Alzheimer's are not in pain.

I hope that if I, too, develop the disease, that I remain grateful and pleasant to others. It is especially hard for caregivers when the patient is mean, yelling, and nasty, which unfortunately happens to some patients. I would hope that no one would force feed me and push food or liquids into my mouth if my mouth was shut. I would not want to be hospitalized in the advanced stages of the disease and would not want to have even a broken bone fixed under those circumstances; just pain control and be allowed to pass on.

Mom was with Dad when he died at 10 a.m. on his eighty-eighth birthday. She had moved his bed into the living room so he could watch what was happening on the street. That morning she found a card stuck in the front door from President Morris of Union College, wishing Dad a happy birthday. Mom went to tell him and he opened his eyes and sang, "Happy birthday to me." Then he closed his eyes and died. It felt like the angels came to take him.

Mom lived to be nearly a hundred years old. At age ninety-seven and a half she moved in with my sister, and before that she was in an independent living facility for older or disabled people. She got shingles at age ninety-seven, and then she got encephalitis from the shingles. You lose your immunity at that age, and I was going out every six weeks or so, for a year, to visit her. She lost her childhood and her old memories, and was left adrift. It's interesting how our past grounds us, even if we're not living in it. Mom was coming out of church with a walker and she fell and broke her hip as she was trying to get into the car. She died within a year of breaking her hip, at age ninety-nine.

Advice for other caregivers

Not everyone has a beautiful death like my father did, but the ambience in the home or assisted living facility makes a huge difference in helping Alzheimer's patients to be more accepting of whatever is happening and to help them be more peaceful and happy. It's important that the patient is in a setting where she/he can feel loved. People who are not supported are more likely to be angry and depressed. They will go in and out cognitively. And sometimes they will have an insight and be totally appropriate, and then that moment will disappear. Always, at some level, that person is still a sentient being.

I have two patients at a memory care home, and the fact that their great grandchildren are able to be in touch with them is a blessing for both the kids and the patients. It's wonderful to have been blessed by a great grandparent. Another woman was just horrible when she came out here to be near her daughter. Her daughter, who had patience and was able to stay strong and not get too depressed by the abuse, converted this woman into a delightful, sweet person. Sometimes it goes the other way. The important thing is to resolve whatever issues you have with your parents. Get rid of resentment and leave all those things behind. Use whatever time you have left to support the main caregiver with love. And, as a caregiver, you want to learn how to connect to the person as a soul. It's important to make that soul connection because there is still a person inside to be respected and honored.

* * *

Julie Carpenter, MD is a family physician who practiced in Boulder County for forty years, initially as a solo practitioner, and then for twenty years as a doctor at Dakota Ridge Family Medicine. She graduated with honors from NYU Medical School and has done volunteer work in Haiti and Tibet, as well as at the People's Clinic at its inception in Boulder County. She loves being outdoors and enjoys hiking, singing, writing, and dance. Email Dr. Carpenter at: julietbeatrice99@icloud.com.

9

Hi Mom, I Love You!

By **Marcus Eckenrode**

I guess we all have a selfish need to be remembered. Why wouldn't Mom remember me? I was her last born, her baby. Every time her eyes opened, she seemed to remember me and know that I was there. It's funny how the mother and son connection never ends — whether it's on this earthly plane or not — and how the sweetness between us is always flowing, as I'm sure it will always be. Maybe that sweetness is the basis of why I believe that she remembered me.

I believe the relationship I have with my mom is multi-layered, consisting of a soul and human connection. Despite her very long and slow goodbye, I'm sure that Mom could remember me on the soul plane, and that her soul wasn't impaired, just her mind. That gave me something to work with, so I applied some of the healing and soul work I had learned in India. When Mom opened her eyes, I would look deeply past her mind and memory into her soul energy and say, "Hi Mom, I love you!" I know she heard me every time.

Mom had quite a journey. We all did. Dad covered for her memory lapses the first couple of years. He took care of her, but didn't let us know the extent of her dementia. They lived in a small town in Ohio where life has more continuity from generation to generation. Even though my brothers and sisters didn't live near our parents, we realized that Mom was going through some changes that weren't just simple 'age' issues.

My parents had been married sixty years and Dad was very traditional. He believed that his job was to take care of his wife and family until 'death do us part.' However, at that time, he didn't completely understand what Alzheimer's is and its effects on the patient and family. His job was to take care of Mom forever. We had to work with him so he could understand what to expect as the disease progressed, and how it would affect his wife.

Mom's journey lasted nine long years. I want to emphasize that, in the same way it takes a village to raise a child, it took the whole family to share in some aspect of caring for Mom and Dad. Caring for an Alzheimer's patient is needed on so many levels that it's impossible for one person to do it all. My siblings and I went through many changes over the years of Mom's decline. At first, it was very uncomfortable reversing the parent-child relationship as our parents' health deteriorated. We shared in their care and supported them and each other with the loving nature that we have as individuals. A combination of our Midwestern upbringing and the unique family dynamics of age order and roles were soon rediscovered after many years of being adults and living away from the family home. It took a while for us to find our way, but everyone had a role to play and no one could have envisioned assuming those duties for nine long years.

As fate would have it, Dad had to go in for a major surgery and could no longer cover up Mom's disease, since his own needs became paramount. The responsibilities of caregiving became overwhelming and I took a sabbatical from my work in California to take care of Mom full-time. I arrived in Ohio at our family home without any understanding of the extent of Mom's condition. I was wholly unprepared for the world I soon found myself in. Living with, and caring for, a loved one suffering from Alzheimer's was much more challenging than I could have ever prepared for.

Unbeknownst to me, I had embarked on a journey into the unknown, that included discovering what this life is about and what really constitutes death. The journey would test my patience, commitment, and the love I was able to give to Mom and to myself. When you're a caregiver for someone who might not even know that you are present, you face challenges that force you to reflect on the meaning of life. Since that person happened to be my mother—the one who gave me this beautiful life and made sacrifices for me—I experienced a wake-up call like never before.

Guilt made me realize that these charged emotions could provide a catalyst for growth and self-reflection. Was I capable of doing the right thing? Was I a good son. . .or not? I finally had the epiphany that my family's need for me to suddenly care for my mother was an opportunity to care for the people who loved me the most, and to pay back that love with dignity. It was no longer about me and my wants and needs. This journey, with its twists and turns, truly tested the gentle perseverance that Mom instilled in my soul and taught with the heartfelt grace of a mother's love.

Despite the progression of her disease, Mom was still cute as a button during the day, but a different person at night during "sundowning." Sundowning is a state of confusion at the end of the day that causes worsening symptoms of moodiness, irritability, and disruption of sleep. My mother became very fastidious in her illness and took great care in preparing her bed for the night. She would methodically fold down the comforter, the blanket, and the sheet, and then plump the pillows. Her nightclothes were carefully laid out on top of the comforter.

After long days as a caregiver, putting her to bed at night was a relief and gave me time to spend a couple of hours by myself. I remember going downstairs and crumpling into a chair in the living room. Inevitably, no more than forty-five minutes after tucking Mom in for the night, I would hear a noise coming from her room. When I went upstairs to check on her, the light would be on, the bed perfectly made, and Mom would be completely dressed! I explained that she had to go back to sleep, but she would protest because she thought she had slept the entire night and that it was morning. I would get her ready for bed again and, to my chagrin, I would hear her up and about an hour later. Instead of being upset, I flashed on our changing parent-child roles and how patient Mom was with me when I was a toddler and didn't want to go to sleep. I was sure she was just as tired as I was then and impatient with my lack of cooperation and understanding. Yet, she would tuck me in and tell me to have sweet dreams and that she loved me. This remembrance made me thankful for the opportunity to re-live those magical bedtime moments, while I secretly hoped that Mom would sleep through the night.

I lived far away from my parents, and my family role evolved into handling the heavy issues with Mom, and then mostly with Dad. Taking away the car and convincing them to move out of their home of fifty years into an assisted care facility was tough. Dad had all his wits about him, along with his contentious nature, which made my new role even more difficult. Despite his protestations, Dad did understand the limitations of his age and I know he appreciated help with his business. But he wasn't an easy man and most days we were locked in a contest of wills over the simplest things. A lot of discussion was focused on Mom's care, as well as her increasing needs. Finally, we discussed how it was becoming problematic for them to continue living together in the same apartment. Luckily, we had made arrangements that, when necessary, Mom would go back to the Memory Care Unit and Dad would stay in their apartment.

Despite my wanting to believe Mom was still cognizant of what was going on around her, I was faced with seeing a loved one in a serious state of failing health and appearance. The experience of watching a once vibrant person transform into someone completely different can be very trying and full of despair. For me, the bottom line riddle of this disease is "what is the person's reality?" Is a memory care person's reality gone or has it changed to something else? Is it our arrogance or ignorance that we may not be able to envision another possibility of their reality changing to something other than the reality of the mind, into something on a much grander scale of knowing? Is it possible that she was there and fully present, but in a different state of awareness? Maybe the person can still see and hear everything and comprehend it all on a completely different level. Maybe she does open her eyes to look at me…recognize me…remember me, to let me know she is there and loves me. Is she communicating to me on a level that needs no words? Is she transitioning from the experiential nature of the mind to the soul incarnate of where she came from and to where she may be headed? Was she teaching us her last lesson of the true nature of this amazing life she blessed us with?

Spiritual people have always had the goal of silencing the mind's chatter. In the Western world, there is nothing greater than the power of our minds and the infinite possibilities that our thoughts can manifest. But in Eastern philosophy, the mind is not always to be believed and is generally thought to not be fully supportive of our overall highest good. In the East, the object is to calm the mind, to quiet the so-called "monkey mind," in order to still our thoughts and let the energies of the Universe flow through us naturally, without the filtering of the mind. In many ways, I looked at Mom's Alzheimer's as somewhat akin to the Eastern teachings of silencing the mind. When the mind becomes silent, the true wisdom and memory of the ages begin to flow.

I pondered the possibility of that happening with Mom. Why did we believe that this silencing of her memory meant that she was not listening to the greater messages and memories of her natural life and her soul life? Are we limited in our thinking that this short time on the planet is the only reality there is? Are our lives nothing more than the memories recorded in our minds of our past experiences, without any acknowledgement of a connection to a higher consciousness of soul memories? Wasn't there a possibility that Mom was actually reawakening to her connection to that Universal consciousness and listening and communicating through her soul, and not just through her brain and language? Can we tune into that connection and truly communicate with each other beyond words? That concept intrigued me, especially after witnessing and understanding the capacity of the soul and its power over the limitations of the mind while I was in India.

What really is the transition of life to death? Is it just the removal of the body, or does the soul need that transition, as well, prior to dropping the body? Are we just flesh and bones, or is there a greater purpose to our lives and a more substantial core of the soul that we have become numb to on our earthly quests? My view of Mom's disease, death, and transition had been undergoing major renovations since studying the ancient teaching and healing techniques in India.

And then the unknown, or the Maya as it is called in India, came into my own life when I was diagnosed with cancer and suddenly my personal and caregiver priorities were brought into question. As shocking as that news was to me, I still had to consider my parents' health issues and their ability to handle such information about their youngest child. How do I tell them? Could they understand? Should I just tell Dad and not Mom? I decided to undergo treatment and not let either of them know.

It was a very tough decision to know that I was truly alone in this life now without the care and loving support of my parents during those times of need. It was certainly an ironic twist that suddenly both my parents and I were now facing life-threatening issues. For me, it became a test of living the fullest day possible and not getting caught up in the 'what-ifs' of the future. While my days were trying with my treatment, I understood that I needed to focus on the positives in my own life while presenting that same perspective to my parents. I understood more intimately how they were facing personal end-of-life issues every day, along with the continual loss of their elderly friends. I was lucky that my cancer went into remission, though my treatment prevented my being with my mother until a couple of days before her passing.

My mother's long journey taught me so much about the need to care for our loved ones and fellow human-beings, and my own mortality and necessary surrender to the fact that all of our lives ultimately end. Does our life and purpose stop with our last breath or does it go on indefinitely, challenging what we believe about life? And more importantly, when, if ever, does it stop…during the advanced stages of Alzheimer's, after death, or maybe never at all?

For caregivers, it doesn't ever really end. Hope springs eternal until the last breath; loving this person out of pure heart and duty. And it is a hard duty for everyone involved. It is difficult to remain mentally, physically, and spiritually motivated, to stay hopeful and 'irrationally positive' as one of my teachers calls it.

But our lives go on with our professions, families, and personal commitments. The memories of the devastation of the disease drift away and are replaced by the vibrant feelings of love and an amazing appreciation for the life and gifts the family shared this time around. We have all been gifted with a greater appreciation and preciousness of the life we've been given and the opportunity of sharing our unique qualities, with no expectations but love. When I look at her photo today, I look into those blue eyes and see her soul and say 'Hi Mom, I Love You!' She tells me she hears me every time!

* * *

Marcus Eckenrode is an ocean scientist in California who works in developing scientific studies to help advance ocean renewable energy projects in Hawaii and on the U.S. west coast. He is a certified Life Coach working with clients during transitional life phases combining Sai Shakti healing techniques he learned in India. His profound experience in helping with the care of his mother has led to volunteer work in Hospice and Veteran homes, where he plays music for patients and their families. marcusananda@gmail.com.

10

Let Your Light Shine

By Reverend **Josephine Falls**

I grew up in Pickens, Mississippi with my great-grandfather, Adam Broadenax, picking cotton on the eighty acres of land that he owned. My great-grandfather lived to 116 years old, and my great-grandmother lived to ninety-six. My parents divorced and when I was ten years old I went to live with my mother and step-father on a plantation where we also picked cotton. We owned horses and raised and slaughtered hogs and cows to eat. My mother canned and had a garden so we had plenty of good food year round. We only had to buy sugar and flour. The ugly things you don't talk about — I never saw the ugly racism.

I walked six or seven miles with other children to go to school. Sometimes I'd cry when I got there because my hands were so cold. I also went to Sunday school at an early age (five through eight), where we learned Bible verses that were printed on cards, since we didn't have books. I was baptized at thirteen.

When I was eighteen years old I married my husband Bennie Will Falls, who was nine years older than I. We owned mules and farmed for five years on rented land, picking cotton, growing corn, and raising chickens, hogs, and cattle. We were not sharecroppers, because you'd have to pay too much. Sharecroppers were allowed to use the land in return for a share of the crop produced. We were, what you call, tenant farmers.

Later, Bennie served in Europe during WWII as a laborer and truck driver. Afterwards, he took the GI Bill and became an automotive mechanic. When I was in school, I loved geography and I had read about the Rocky Mountains. When he was in the service, Bennie had been stationed in Pueblo, Colorado. When I met Bennie and we were still dating, something came up about the Rocky Mountains. Bennie said to me, "Jo, the Rocky Mountains are so beautiful, and if you marry me, we will move to Colorado so you can see them every day." We were saved in the Baptist church in Pickens,

Mississippi, but the Lord saw fit to bring us to Colorado. Bennie arrived in November 1951, and I arrived, pregnant with our fourth child, on the ninth of January 1952 on a beautiful day, with our three children, Bennie Junior, Myra, and Robert. And here I still am.

We had four girls and six boys and raised nine of them in this home. All nine graduated from high school and most of them went to college. Three of my sons, Larry, John, and Bennie Junior, have died since 1960, and a baby, Robert Lewis, died at three weeks old in 1948. My daughter Parthenia died at age sixty-one in 2013. But the Lord has been good to me. My five children Myra, Robert, Gloria, Rose, and David are still alive. I have thirteen grandchildren and I don't know exactly how many great grandchildren I have.

After moving to Colorado, I joined the Bethel Church of Christ Holiness in Denver and became a deaconess of the church. Deacon means servant. I helped prepare and attend to the Holy Sacraments, such as baptism and Holy Communion. My husband was a deacon and helped with the finances for more than thirty-three years.

Bennie was in his fifties when he started showing memory loss. In 1972, we went to Omaha, Nebraska for a church convention and I noticed that he couldn't hold a conversation. He started having seizures, but he was well enough to drive back to Denver. He got progressively worse and started falling off the bed at night. I finally got him to go to the hospital and he was diagnosed, first with seizures, and then with Alzheimer's when he was only fifty-five. Sometimes he'd leave the house and not come home until 5a.m. I'd ask, "Where have you been?" He'd say, "I was downtown," but I knew that he had gotten lost.

Then my son Larry got colon cancer. I was working for the Department of Revenue at the time. The doctor said, "Mrs. Falls, Larry isn't sick enough to be in the hospital, but I want a nice place for him." I prayed and then I said, "I'll take him home and take care of him." So I gave up my job and took care of my son. It made me stronger in my faith. As my husband got sicker, he got depressed and thought I was giving too much attention to my son. Bennie started going in and out of the hospital. Then Larry passed away in 1982. He was only twenty-six. I kept the faith. It was hard, but my Lord gave me strength. The only time my faith in God wavered was when my mother was murdered in 1959.

One day Bennie came to bed with a butcher's knife. He dropped it when he was taking off his clothes. He didn't move into the nursing home right then. Instead, they put him on medication. Finally, my grandson told his momma that Grandpa was throwing away his pills, and his mother told me. I had fear, but I didn't show it. I stayed watchful. "Watch and pray," the Bible says. For many nights I couldn't sleep. I cared for him the whole time he was getting worse, and then finally in 1985, he went into a nursing home because he stopped taking his medication and I couldn't take care of him anymore.

While all this was happening, I was ordained as a reverend and became a licensed, ordained minister. I knew the Lord had called me into the ministry, so I went to my pastor and told him that the Lord called me. He said, "I can't ordain a woman." So the Lord let me know that I had to be humble. I did a three-year ministry at a nursing home and never missed a Sunday. Again, I went to the pastor and told him that I knew I'd been called to the ministry. Again he said, "I can't ordain you."

The Holy Spirit came through and told me to go to Mt. Gilead Baptist Church where I could exercise my gift. I went there and they had a minister's school that I attended. I had been a missionary and evangelist. When it came time for the other students to get ordained, I was sitting in the back of the church shaking. The pastor looked at me and said, "Why are you sitting back there?" So I went up and they tested me. I have no idea how I answered those questions, because the other six or seven people who were getting ordained had been in classes for a year and I had only been in classes for two months. But the reverend said, "Let's ordain Sister Falls so she can stop bootlegging the Gospel and do it legally."

I was ordained on Super Bowl Sunday in 1987 and gained the title Reverend Josephine Falls. Once ordained, we can automatically be called reverend because we reverence the Lord. I'm also a pastor — a leader of the flock — because I have a congregation and I do evangelistic work in the world. The next step was to start preaching.

In 1989, a pastor that was looking for a pastor to replace him, because the Lord said to him that he should do outreach work, asked me to preach every Sunday. He didn't have a church, so I said, "I don't have a mansion, but I'm willing to bring the church to my home." I knew he wasn't looking for a woman, but I have been preaching ever since. I've also been a chaplain with the Denver Police Department for the past twenty-nine years, and served as chaplain for the Greater Metro Denver Ministerial Alliance for over ten years. I'm eighty-seven years old and I've worked all my life—picking cotton, farming, as a CNA (certified nursing assistant), and for the Colorado Department of Revenue, the Colorado Department of Youth Services, and the School of Nursing at University of Colorado Hospital. I worked at the First National Bank of Denver for eight and a half years, and I've also been an election judge for over twenty-five years.

I worked the whole time Bennie was sick. We were married over forty-eight years and he knew us all until the end. He died at the age of seventy-five in 1994, the Sunday after Thanksgiving. I miss Bennie, but I have the ministry. Every Sunday I have a Sunday school at 9 a.m. and a worship service at 11 a.m. My daughter teaches, a member plays the piano, and my son is a deacon. I typically get thirty-five people, and sometimes just eight or nine. I love the work because I love people! Most of all I love Jesus Christ!

Several years ago I was on the bus on my way home from work when the Lord spoke to me through the Holy Spirit and said, "A great door is open to you." It scared me. I came home and started looking up scriptures. The Lord was telling me that many opportunities were coming to me. Since then, I've traveled to many states in the U.S. and to Canada. I went to Israel in 2006, where I spent ten days in Jerusalem and got baptized in the Jordon River. In 2011, I went to South Korea with one hundred and seventy-two pastors. It was awesome.

I'm healthy, besides having diabetes. I just thank the Lord and keep on going. I have the ministry and I'm an election judge and a chaplain for the International Conference of Police Chaplains (ICPC) in the Denver police department. I still reach out to people because of my faith in the Lord. I say, "Lord, I thank you for my life, health, and strength, and most of all for you, Jesus, for being in my life."

Most of all, you have to be saved and know the Lord, accept the Lord, and realize we need our savior. Acknowledge that and ask the Lord to come into your life. If you believe it, you have to cultivate it. Believe the word and act on the word. When I read the Bible, I believe the Lord. Be encouraged. You are here to help somebody else. Be strong. Be courageous. Praise God. He will do what you ask Him. We have to ask the Lord for forgiveness. Leave behind all the worldly stuff and let your light shine.

* * *

*Reverend **Josephine Falls** is a beloved community member of Denver, Colorado, where she has lived since 1952. She and her late husband Bennie had ten children; a baby boy died in infancy, and three sons have died since 1960. Her daughter Parthenia died at age sixty-one in 2013. Reverend Falls has five living children, thirteen grandchildren and many great grandchildren. She was ordained as a Baptist minister in 1987 and became a pastor shortly thereafter. She has been offering services in her home since 1991. She can be reached at: 303-296-2575.*

11

Connected by Spirit

By **Cindy Jackson**

My mom, Zona Allred, was diagnosed with Alzheimer's at seventy years old. But she had problems for two to three years before that, which made things difficult for her. Mom was one quarter Native American, (Cree or Creek, we're not sure), and she lived most of her life in Texas. She and my dad divorced when I was in high school. One year after my marriage, I moved to Virginia. Mom stayed in Texas to be near my brother, my sister, and her own siblings. About seven years later, my younger sister moved to Maryland. Later, when I invited Mom to move closer to me, she wouldn't move because she still wanted to help my brother. He lived with Mom, off and on, for several years. When he got married in 2003, he lived six blocks away from her.

Mom worked in retail for five or six years, and worked for her church another five or six years. After she retired from retail, she was a pre-school teacher until her first grandson, my brother's child, was born. By the time she started taking care of her grandson in 2004, she was showing some signs of short-term memory loss and confusion. She couldn't keep the thermostat adjusted properly for the seasons and she said weird things like, "The hot water is out," even though my brother had just checked the tank and adjusted the temperature setting for her. It turned out she would leave the faucets on when she left the room.

My brother took Mom to the doctor and found she had lost most of the vision in one eye and had hearing loss. Drops for her eye pressure and hearing aids helped a little, but finally my brother took her to be evaluated for dementia. Over this time period, I could only go and visit her four to seven days at a time. Mom was pretty good at hiding her memory loss and other difficulties. She soon lost the skills she needed to cook, and she became depressed when my brother wouldn't let her take care of his son any longer because of the safety issues for both of them. Her physician was able to get a home health care nurse to come out once a week for a few hours, but it really wasn't enough contact for her.

In 2008, my brother, who had been visiting her every morning to give her the recommended supplements and prescriptions, needed a break from his caregiving and was going to be gone for several days and no one else was available to help her. We all knew she would soon need more constant care. I had been looking at the options near me, since there wasn't a subsidized assisted living available with memory care anywhere near where my brother lived.

While my brother was away, Mom came to visit me and my husband and son in Virginia, for what we thought would be three weeks. While she was with us, she got a scratch on her leg that became badly infected with cellulitis (a bacterial infection in the tissues beneath the skin). We couldn't let her go home since her doctor wouldn't approve full day care for when my brother was going to be away, and there was no follow-up appointment available to make sure the antibiotic was effective. My husband and I decided to just keep her with us, ready or not. I had hoped to have my home arranged so she could spend weekends with us when she was in her own room at the assisted living community.

We have a two-bedroom house and our son was four years old at the time, plus I ran a home pre-school. I thought Mom could be helpful, but she wasn't able to do much in the house except hang clothes on the line and fold them. She'd hover around the kids and disrupt their play, even though she was trying to be helpful. We had an outdoor-based program and one day she ended up in a tug-of-war with my son Barun. She hit him and he was devastated. The incident was a real wake-up call for me, and I realized it might not work to have Mom in the house for an extended period of time.

My family was camping out in the basement and we had to be vigilant because Mom was a wanderer. And four-year-old Barun often had to be her guide, directing her from point A to point B. We had to take care of Mom 24/7 and the interactions between her and my son got hard since she couldn't understand he was more capable than the two year olds she was used to taking care of. It was especially difficult when I was caught in the middle, trying to do the right thing for both of them at the same time.

John, my husband, saw how worried I was about Mom going back to Texas. We didn't know how long we'd be able to take care of her at home. He took over a lot of the responsibility caring for our son and the house, as well as looking out for Mom, when I needed to be with our son or just rest. I was running the pre-school and had to stay up late doing legal paper work to transfer her bank accounts, social security, and Medicare from Texas to Virginia. The only way she would be able to go into assisted living was to sell her house, so I had to go through the legal process to become her guardian and conservator.

Mom ended up living with us for six months, since I was the only family member who was available to care for her full-time. Even though it was challenging at times, it was so good to have her here and connect with her for that time. I went to Alzheimer's support groups, and Mom and my son and I also attended a group support program together.

John devoted himself to helping manage our household. He told me, "I don't want you to get sick," and encouraged me to have time to myself. I took Mom to a gym program for seniors, and I worked out while she was doing a little exercise. Thanks to John, I was also able to do some of the things I love to do three to four times a month, and I went to Zero Balancing workshops so I could re-establish my bodywork practice that had gone on hold when we adopted our son.

I knew that I had to find an assisted care home for Mom. In Texas, she had been a country girl who climbed fences and loved walking in open spaces. We live on six acres with a pond and creek, and now she was a wanderer. I worried that she would get lost and hurt in the woods surrounding our property. We found a beautiful memory care home in town called Our Lady of Peace, which was established by the Catholic Diocese of Richmond, one of the oldest dioceses in the country.

Mom had a private room for one year and then a compatible room-mate for the next year and a half. It was a good situation. Mom thought most of the residents were distant relatives and was help-ful to the friends who had less mobility than she did. The facility had a wonderful activities program and there was a playground within walking distance so Barun, Mom, and I could go on outings together. Best of all, having Mom live there, let me be a mom again. The free time also allowed me to serve my mother in emotional and spiritual ways since I didn't have to care for her daily needs.

Zona was a devout Christian. Even though I had not been involved in a church for a long time and was studying Buddhism, we were able to grow closer spiritually as she lost some of her theological concepts. I found that, because my Buddhist practices focused on awareness and loving kindness, I had more understanding and patience with Mom. I was able to communicate the core beliefs that are the same in Christianity and Buddhism — love, compassion, and forgiveness. I was also able to utilize my background as an early-childhood educator to understand where Mom was going developmentally. Maybe you've heard the phrase "growing down." Rather than growing up with new abilities, people with dementia go backwards in developmental stages. I relied on my professional knowledge and Buddhist practices to understand that Mom's mental age and emotional behavior were no reflection on what I was doing.

A basic belief in Buddhism is seeing all people as your mother, and so I saw that her suffering was the same as what other "mothers" in my life were going through. Of course, she had her own karmic destiny. The things she developed in her life, like enjoying nature, friendliness, playfulness, empathy, and deep heartfelt trust in Christ, were still serving her well, but I knew she didn't have the capacity to heal some of her emotional wounds she hadn't dealt with before Alzheimer's.

I made a practice of saying this prayer offering compassion: "All are my mothers and have been my mothers primordially. I have compassion for each of the sentient beings, the mothers who experience infinite sufferings…May everyone purify their misunderstandings, accumulate virtues, and may we all gain these benefits." I have said this daily for many years, but seeing it so directly with Mom, it helped me be more at peace as I watched her slowly decline; especially in the last three or four months when her physical health was declining along with increasing dementia.

Mom was able to go with us to our meditation center a few times and our lamas (Tibetan teachers) greeted her. Those visits brought out the best in her. Her loving nature shone beautifully and I was able to see underneath the Alzheimer's diagnosis and who she really was—a kind, loving, radiant person.

One time, when Mom was doing so poorly, one of the lamas came to visit her at her memory care facility. I had contacted hospice, as she was eating and drinking very little and refused to take her medicine and supplements. She had only met the lama once, but she lit up and latched onto him, saying she remembered him. She held his hand for a long time and she listened carefully when he reminded her to connect with her heart. He said a few blessings and brought her flowers and some water imbued with prayers during a special meditation practice he did. She began feeling better over the next couple of days and was released from hospice care in a couple of weeks.

The spirituality she instilled in me when I was a child—faith, love, gratitude, and compassion—was what connected us as her mental capacity decreased. I found it fascinating that, despite our having different practices, we both seemed to understand each other better. And I felt closer to Mom as our verbal communication gave way to more heart communication, hugs, hand holding, and laughter at my son.

When I visited her without Barun, I was able to share breathing practices with her which clarify the mind and are healing to the body. We'd sit together and inhale and exhale deeply which slows the breathing and increases oxygenation to the brain and body. Sometimes friends offered complementary therapies such as cranial sacral therapy, which she enjoyed. She got Body Talk treatments—a gentle type of energy healing that uses muscle testing and the body's natural wisdom to locate weakened lines of communication within the body.

I am a Zero Balancing practitioner and applied my training of integrating the deepest flows of energy through bones and joints for Mom's whole body. She was able to put my hand where she felt pain or stiffness, and I applied light pressure and traction to the bones and ligaments. This technique reduces pain, and helps one to relax, feel more alert, calm, and peaceful. It also improves overall functioning. After any one of these treatments, Mom could pull her inner resources together for up to a week. The treatments always cleared her disorientation.

As Barun got older, it became more difficult for him to connect with his grandma. As Mom declined, it got harder for me as well. When I finally was able to let go of my guilt feelings of not being able to do more for her and realize that the Alzheimer's was ultimately Mom's experience of what she brought into this life, I was able to relax and give her love and feel joy just by being with her.

One day I went in to the home to tell her that I'd be going on a trip for a week and wouldn't see her. She responded by saying, "Now, honey, I want you to take good care of yourself and have a good time." In that moment, I felt her become my mom again for the first time in about five years. And I knew from our communication that she was my mother and loved me.

I experienced much less trauma at Mom's death than others I've spoken with, because we lost her incrementally over such a long period of time. My siblings and I had also been able to agree that we didn't want to prolong her life any more than what was natural. And each of us let her know, in our own way, that when she was ready, she should go to join Jesus to get her heavenly reward. She died at age seventy-eight having spent less than a week in a wheelchair.

Healing therapies my friends and I used with Zona Allred:

- Body Talk is a simple, safe, effective system of integrative health care. It is a holistic approach to healing, based on proven principles of energy medicine. Body Talk helps synchronize the body's natural functions to achieve and maintain healing and growth on all levels—physical, emotional, mental, and spiritual.

- Cranial sacral therapy involves a light pressure applied to the head, along the spine, all the way to the sacrum in a prescribed way, in order to alleviate stress and correct imbalances in the central nervous system.

- Zero Balancing was developed by Dr. Fritz Smith in the early 1970s from his practice of osteopathy and acupuncture. It is a non-diagnostic system done through clothing that focuses on our body's capacity to return to well-being. Zero Balancers use gentle traction and direct pressure with an awareness of each person's individual pattern of bone and joint tension. The protocol addresses the major joints and the full spine, allowing the whole person to deeply relax. www.zerobalancing.com

• Breathing practices from Tibetan yoga

* * *

Cindy Allred-Jackson *has degrees in photography and education, and a professional certificate and teaching credential in Zero Balancing. In 1985, she and her husband traveled around the world. It was on that trip that she connected with Tibetan Buddhism in Nepal. Cindy has taught in Charlottesville, Virginia City Schools, and Charlottesville Waldorf School, and has owned a home pre-school. She currently has a private Zero Balancing practice near downtown Charlottesville and continues to study wellness-based therapies. She lives on six hilly acres with her husband and son near the Blue Ridge Mountains. Contact Cindy at* yeshemama@gmail.com *or* wholebody-wellbeing.com. *Follow her at:* wholebodywellbeing.wordpress.com.

12

Be Still

By **Graham Kolb**

I was a single, married caregiver with a Younger Onset Alzheimer's spouse. My wife Kaki (nickname for Catherine) was diagnosed in January 2006, at age fifty-eight, with Alzheimer's disease. We were both professionals. She had degrees in elementary education, computer science, and accounting and eventually became a CPA with her own business. I worked for the Department of Defense in their health care agency and was in charge of the technical requirements for multibillion-dollar contracts. I was also a team leader for the evaluation of the technical requirements of the procurements.

We were both breadwinners in our family, although we could not have children. In our forty plus years of marriage, she handled the 'big stuff' (financial planning, investments, and legal issues) and I took care of the 'operational stuff' such as paying the bills, bookkeeping, and running the household. Since I was the neat one, I took care of most of the household duties and, of course, the upkeep of the house and yard. So I was already the domestic one. But Kaki had her herb garden and made most of the decisions on the house decor.

So when Kaki was diagnosed, I was already carrying most of the household load. Buying a new car helped solve the problem of getting Kaki to stop driving, since she couldn't figure out how to start it. But this added to my duties of making sure she got to her appointments (doctor, hairdresser) while I was still working. Venturing into unfamiliar territory, I finally took over the management of our financial investments.

The biggest change for me in the daily routine was to start cooking. Kaki was an excellent cook who got me interested in the culinary art. At one time, we had over three hundred and eighty cookbooks which she read like novels. We enjoyed cooking together and going to cooking classes. One of our fondest memories was eating at the Cooking Institute of America in California where we both separately ate a meal for two! The staff was amazed. And then we had dessert!

These marriage duties had been worked out over our long marriage and we were comfortable with our roles. We were just beginning to enjoy life with more disposable income. We joined a timeshare, which forced us to finally take great vacations. Then I noticed that Kaki began to withdraw from activities. I didn't realize what was happening until about nine months before the diagnosis, when I thought she should see her doctor for depression.

The biggest challenge with the diagnosis was that we no longer could make decisions as partners. I gradually had to assume the role as the sole decision maker, sometimes playing the bad guy who wouldn't allow Kaki to drive or cook anymore. It was so hard. After all those years of togetherness, I was alone.

I've been asked, "What was the most challenging part of caring for your wife?" Initially, it was keeping her safe and physically healthy. Even though she was in a secure Alzheimer's facility the final year of her life, that feeling of concern never diminished. It was also hard watching Kaki die a little every day; watching a bright mind being wasted little by little. Eventually, she wasn't able to recall my name, even though she still told me that she loved me. Probably the worst thing was to lose the loving, caring relationship I had with the person I planned to spend the 'golden years' with. This was not what I dreamed of for retirement.

Initially, Kaki didn't want anyone to know about the diagnosis, although some people close to us already knew something was wrong. After telling the family and friends, we got help from the Alzheimer's Association by attending the Early (now called Younger) Onset Support Group. That was so wonderful and supportive. After about one and a half years, I took the Savvy Caregiver Class, which gave me a greater insight into caring for my wife.

Then, after a very long dry spell, Kaki and I rejoined the Episcopal Church. The liturgy, music, and friendship were wonderful for helping to lift her up for awhile. (She and I had been long-time Episcopalians and her grandfather had been a priest.) Being with new friends and fellowship was a huge help to me. I joined the Men's Thursday Fellowship group and was assigned a Stephen

Lay Minister*, whom I met with on a weekly basis for five years. Our meetings helped me keep an even keel.

Prior to placing Kaki in a memory care home, and while I was still working, I took her to the Johnson Center in Denver once a week for field trips and company, until she refused to go anymore. As Kaki's dementia progressed and I was forced to retire in January 2008, she became more and more unmanageable. I engaged an agency that was familiar with Alzheimer's and began to have in-home care for Kaki, so I could do chores and have some time to myself.

In April 2010 when the drugs could not control her and she began hitting the caregivers and trying to wander away, I placed her in a memory care facility. I began looking at facilities six months prior to the move because I knew this day was coming. Because I took time searching for a memory care home for Kaki before an emergency situation arose, I was able to make a rational decision based on facts and was not pressured to make an uninformed decision.

Throughout this, one individual was God-sent. Even though she was an employee of the home care agency, she stuck with us for two and half years and continued to visit and watch over Kaki. Although the facility was full of wonderful caregivers, you still have to advocate for your loved one. I went as much as possible to oversee Kaki's care and provide love, even after she was put on hospice care.

Towards the end of the disease, Kaki weighed less than eighty pounds. She had three falls with head injuries in eight months, and developed a blood clot on the brain. The last fall caused a stroke, which affected her left side, so she wasn't allowed to walk without help. She was watched closely since she was unable to stand without assistance. Although she was still eating, she was very weak and was not retaining any weight. She died July 31, 2013.

If you have a loved one with Alzheimer's, I recommend that you seek support where you can find it; be it family, friends, church, or associations. Accept the kindness of others and be open to receiving help from strangers. Take time for yourself, be alone to grieve, but also be active —take walks, join a gym, play golf, or bike with friends. Take care of yourself, for this is truly the long goodbye. Interestingly, in a period of two weeks, various people reminded me via scripture, posters, and in news articles, to just *be still*. I am now at peace with the final outcome as there is nothing further I can do. "Be still and know that I am God" (Psalm 46:10). Take care of yourself. Be still.

*Stephen Ministry consists of trained and supervised laypersons called Stephen Ministers, who provide support and Christian care to individuals facing life challenges.

* * *

Graham Kolb *went to Northeast Louisiana State College (NLSC) where he met his wife, Catherine (Kaki). They got married after graduation and Graham entered the U.S. Army for a two-year reserve commitment. Graham went on to receive an M.S. in biology and they moved to Colorado, where he went to work for the Department of the Army's Mycobacterium Lab (TB) while Kaki worked for the Girl Scouts. He switched jobs to work for the Department of Defense, OCHAMPUS (now called TRICARE), providing health care benefits and services to members of the Armed Services. Graham spent thirty-five years working for the Federal Government before retiring in 2008 to take care of Kaki. Reach Graham at:* grahamkolb@comcast.net.

13

In Loving Memory

By **Doshin Michael Nelson**

My mother was a devout Catholic and never forgave me for becoming a Buddhist priest instead of a Catholic priest. From her perspective, she thought I was a heathen. She didn't think there were other ways to find God. That was the baggage we carried into the arrival of her onset of Alzheimer's.

I had taken the Boddhisatva vows to serve all sentient and insentient beings until every blade of grass is awake, which is a very long time—an inconceivable amount of time. It was shortly after I dedicated my life to service that my service assignment appeared. I got a phone call that my mother, age eighty-five, had fallen and was unable to get up. I immediately drove five hours to Monte Vista, Colorado—an isolated farming community where she was in the hospital, and where I grew up. After repeated x-rays and MRIs, the doctors found that my mother had a ruptured disc. They put her on a Flight for Life® Colorado helicopter and flew her to Swedish hospital in Denver. She was in considerable pain and very medicated.

It became clear that, since I was the only direct relative, I'd have to make the decision about what type of treatment was appropriate. My mother had extremely good insurance, so cost was not a problem. In fact, today you can't get the type of insurance she had. After everything she went through, she only had to pay fifty dollars out of pocket. It became apparent that she had to have surgery to repair the ruptured disc, or she'd never be able to walk again.

Mother endured a five to seven hour operation, and when she came out of it, her memory was gone. Previously, she had been living independently with very mild cognitive impairment, while maintaining a five-acre garden and supplying all the flowers to the church. After the surgery, her memory loss increased to full-blown dementia. Her long-term memory was intact, but her short-term memory was gone. Most of the time, she remembered who I was.

But one minute after eating breakfast, she couldn't remember that she had eaten breakfast, so she would think that she was hungry again.

There was no doubt in my mind whom I needed to serve. It appeared serendipitously in my life, and caring for my mother was an extremely healing event for me because of the openness and the willingness with which I was committed to offer my service. If my mother had needed me another time in my life, I would have been too busy or too resistant. The actual timing of her illness turned out to be a great gift for her and for me.

After my mother spent several months at a rehab facility and then at a nursing home, it was time for me to make the decision of whether to leave her in a rest home or take her home. The insurance would have paid for the rest home, but that wasn't the issue. I realized there was only one thing to do— after I dropped into silence and looked at the situation from pure awareness— and that was to take Mother home where I could provide full-time care.

When the nursing home care team heard of my decision, they sat me down and told me that I was crazy because it would take three full-time people to care for my mother. I listened to their arguments, which were quite logical, and thanked them for their insights. They didn't realize that I had totally committed my life to service and that my service had just appeared. So I took Mother home and cared for her.

I was fortunate because our situation wasn't like the stories that I'd heard from other people who became full-time caregivers. Mother's long-term memory was there, and because I came to live in the house where she'd always lived, she regained some basic functionality. Everything was very familiar to her. Had I taken her out of that house, it would have been a disaster.

When Mother physically recovered from the back surgery, she was able to do self-care things, such as brushing her teeth and bathing. However, she needed help remembering what, how, and when to do those things. But she couldn't cook, do laundry, or any of the things she'd always done. She'd get so mad and frustrated, and she'd complain, "My memory used to be so good and now I can't remember anything." After about six months, I had to take care of her personal hygiene, and someone always had to be there with her.

The situation was quite interesting because I was married at the time. Our son had left the nest, and the same day that I went to Monte Verde to see what was wrong with Mother, my wife got a call that her mother was ill in California. She went to care for her mother, who died a month later, and I ended up caring for my mother and living with her for two years. My wife would come visit us every month or so. This shared experience of caring for our mothers bonded us together in a way that is indescribable. There was an understanding that this was the right thing to do. Although it created space in our lives, it brought us close together through the deep caring that we were doing.

I observed that this two-year period was a time of a deepening of spirit for my mother. God is kind — in that we lose the memory of the things that keep us from walking the spiritual journey that we must take when we die. Joan Halifax, a Zen Buddhist roshi, author, and the founder of *Project on Being with Dying,* said that in order to die peacefully, we will all be called to let go of everything. What I noticed with my mother was that she was holding some deep resentments about the people she loved: me, because I'd been such a rebellious child; my father, because he had a drinking problem that deeply affected her life; and her father.

My mother's father was German and very authoritarian. He believed that women didn't need an education past eighth grade. Mother had to drop out of school because of him. She never forgave him for that, yet she never rebelled against him. People would come to visit and listen out of kindness as Mother repeated the same story over and over about how her father made her drop out of school. She had held onto this resentment. As she was nearing death, she first forgave me for being such a rascal of a son. Then she forgave my father for his drinking and measuring his life out with coffee spoons. And finally, she forgave her father for being a patriarchal authoritarian that robbed her of the right to an education. At the very end, she forgave herself.

My mother was able to do this with my help. This was my service as the Zen priest; offering gentle, loving kindness, spiritual direction, and deep shadow work. The anger and the part of my mother's personality that resented her father and the other males in her family had been disowned and pushed into the shadows. She had to reclaim this disowned self and make friends with it. I was able to gently help her with this process; of bringing this part of her out of the shadows into the light of conscious awareness in order to find liberation. It is not the truth, but this kind of truthfulness that sets us free.

My teacher, Jun Po, Roshi the Abbot of the Hollow Bones Order of Rinzai Zen (in which I'm also a lineage holder and Zen Master) told me that the only problem with Zen and psychotherapy is that they don't work. I really find that to be true because psychotherapy deals in the realm of the ego. It's about how to adapt the ego to the insanity of a specific culture. Zen is a path of selfless awareness, of transcending the ego and seeing through the delusion of the permanent self.

Author and Integral theorist Ken Wilbur says Zen is about waking up and enlightenment is waking up and growing up. Zen helps you wake up, but it doesn't help you grow up. Psychotherapy helps you grow up, but it doesn't help you wake up. The two together — Zen dealing with absolute mind and psychotherapy dealing with relative mind — are required in order to be fully functional, liberated, and free.

So what I was doing was helping my mother grow up and deal with the wounding that she'd been carrying all her life. I was helping her come to terms with the way she was victimized, which enabled her to forgive herself for not taking responsibility for her own education, which she could have done later in life. I was helping her wake up. I was helping her find the peace that is always already here in this moment. I loved her and accepted her for who she was in the moment. I didn't try to change her. I didn't co-enable the stories she'd been telling herself for years. I kept pointing to the deeper truth of who she was beyond her stories and the resentments, which she was unaware of.

There's a Jesuit priest named Anthon DiMello, an Indian man from Calcutta, who is one of my favorite teachers. He was quite awake, and he said something that really touched me.

"Our deepest longing as human beings is for unity with God."

"And how do you attain unity with God ?" you ask.

His answer was "silence."

"What is silence?" you ask.

His answer is "meditation."

"And what is meditation?" you ask.

His answer was "silence."

So I would go into the garden with my mother and tend to what was left of the flowers, and she would sit there and meditate. She would just sit in the silence; or as Father Thomas Keating, another Catholic priest who is as awake as a Zen master, would say, "Sitting in the Grace of God." Father Thomas Keating would use the word "sitting" figuratively when talking about sitting in the grace of God.

I'm a Zen guy and we don't use the word God because it carries too much baggage. We use the word Samadhi, which means *unreasonable joy*. It's the joy that comes for no reason. No one can give you this joy and no one can take it away. It's the joy that comes when you touch the deep truth of who you are, or when you touch the ineffable silence — this purity of meditative mind. So what I did was to teach my mother how to meditate. Not anything at all like teaching someone else as a Zen master, but by sitting with her in the garden in the Grace of God — in Samadhi and transmitting the eloquent silence of this mind to her.

In the two years I cared for my mother, I set boundaries by making time for my own spiritual practice. I made time to meditate and I meditated more than I regularly would. I needed the deep spiritual awareness of who I really am, in order to keep from falling into the shallow self-pity of 'poor me' the caregiver. I needed the spiritual practice of continually witnessing everything arising in my experience, in order to not fall victim to the part of myself that makes excuses about why I can't do the one right thing there is to do. It's only in silence — in purity of awareness beyond thought, feeling, and self-referencing mind — that we are able to discern the one right thing to do. Once we see what it is, then we come up to this deep caring, which is the essence of what makes us human. It's that type of caring which moves us to run into a burning building to save a dog without any thought of our own safety. We come up from silent witnessing to this deep place of selfless caring and execute the "one right thing to do" that we have seen from the silent empty mind.

Caring for my mother with deep clarity and compassion was the spiritual practice that I had to continually practice. That was the boundary I set for myself. I would not allow my whining little ego any space to speak. This simple boundary enabled me to be of service to my mother until I finally saw that we were not separate; that our lives were deeply intertwined and inter-connected. I realized that in serving her, I was serving all beings and truly serving myself. She was modeling for me how to forgive everyone that I resented, and how the karma of my own internal resentment was blocking my own insight and liberation. It was a great gift.

Momma took me back to "school" and helped me develop patience and the capacity for compassion and forgiveness that paved the way to my own liberation. Now there's room for everything — tears, joy, sadness, and especially the deep gratitude. May all of you be so blessed as to have such a great teacher at such a perfect time.

In gratitude and service,

Rev. Doshin Michael Nelson, Roshi

* * *

Doshin Michael Nelson is a Buddhist priest and Zen Master. He cared full-time for his mother, who lapsed into full-blown disabling dementia after undergoing a surgical procedure. He believes it is necessary to take a three-pronged approach to caregiving. First, at the beginning, because caregiving for someone with dementia is like having three full-time jobs, it's important to develop a healthy view that will not block your insight or make the act self-defeating. Second, when you're in the thick of things, make sure you take care of yourself and set boundaries so you can stay healthy. And, finally, after your loved one has passed, reflect deeply on the experience so you are able to see the wisdom that comes out of it. Doshin Nelson can be reached at: <u>doshin@integralzen.org</u> *and* <u>www.integralzen.org</u>.

14

The Greatest Generation and Alzheimer's

By **Dan Thomas**

My dad was a member of what Tom Brokaw used as the title of his wonderful 1998 book, *The Greatest Generation*. My dad passed away from Alzheimer's in 1992 in Washington, D.C. at the age of eighty-one. He was born and raised in Tennessee where his father lost everything during the Depression. When Dad was in his early twenties, he ventured north in search of work. Eventually, he was successful in landing a job with GMAC (the Finance arm of General Motors) in Washington, D.C. as a "repo man" — that wonderful person who goes out in the field to repossess cars from people who defaulted on their car loans.

Dad met my mother through friends in D.C. and they were married on May 3, 1941. Seven months after their wedding, the world changed with the attack on Pearl Harbor. Like many, rather than wait to be drafted, Dad enlisted in the Army and was selected to go through the intense Officer Candidate School (OCS). After six weeks, he graduated as a First Lieutenant Ordnance officer. I still have his notebook from OCS that reflects how times have changed. In the section on chemical warfare, specifically:

"Defending Against Lung Irritants," his entry reads "… to test for lung irritant – smoke a cigarette and if metallic taste is obtained – gas has been breathed." The notes went on to document the use of gas masks.

After his training, Dad was deployed to Europe from 1942 to 1945 as part of the First Army. He served in Iceland and England before taking part in the Normandy invasion (D-Day) in June 1944, and in the Battle of the Bulge a few months later. Interestingly, he took many pictures while serving and meticulously wrote notes on the back of them, which provide some terrific insight into the thoughts of a soldier in World War II.

When Dad passed away, I went through the cardboard boxes in his basement that contained all these pictures and took many of them and had them framed and labeled with his notes on the back. Some of the most interesting are from August 1945, shortly after the U.S. Army occupied Berlin. One of the most amazing photos was of Hitler's destroyed office, which he labeled "- this is Hitler's desk- kaput!" In addition to the interesting pictures, there was a five-page, handwritten letter to my mother dated August 2, 1945 — on Hitler's personal stationery! It also had at the top #530 — which I am guessing was the number of letters he sent to my mother at that point of his three-year deployment.

One part of his letter included a description of what he was seeing in Berlin at that time. "The city is really beat up in the center, but on the outskirts it isn't quite as bad. The people are in pretty sad shape and are beginning to look quite hungry. Their sole occupation now is to look for food and that is the way they spend their time. They eat every scrap of food that the soldiers throw away, and that situation is true all over Germany. At our own mess hall, the civilians line up at the garbage can and carry off everything the G.I.s don't eat. They take coffee grounds and dry them out to make coffee, and repeat the process two or three times." He signed the letter with "I love you, baby and someday soon I'll see you – all yours 'till Germany conquers the world.'"

WOW. I guess he looked at the civilians as victims of Hitler's terror too. Of course, like many of the Greatest Generation, he never talked about the war because he considered his time in the army as "just doing my job."

After the war, Dad returned to D.C. and his job at GMAC, and there were good times for the country. From 1946 until his retirement from GMAC in 1972, (remember when you worked for one company for your entire career?) he steadily progressed in management and had a good career. After his retirement, he and my mother enjoyed about fifteen years of traveling, grandkids, and life, until *things* began to change in the late 1980s. Those *things* were the beginning of the Alzheimer's journey for all of us.

Even though my father was an astute finance guy, he asked me to review his tax returns starting in the late 1970s. I was a CPA and happy to review his relatively straight forward returns. I reviewed them year after year, and they were always perfect — until *things* changed. In 1987, I opened his return file and there was only one number on the page and it was not correct. It was essentially a blank return. At age seventy-six, he could no longer comprehend financial matters that he had done so well his entire life. It was one of the saddest days in my life.

My mother, who was five years younger than my father and in okay health, became the primary caregiver. My wife became the support and backup to my mother. We were not entirely surprised about his failing because his older brother passed away ten years prior (about 1977) with what, in those days, was called dementia. My mother was a typical housewife of the fifties and sixties and had great common sense, but no financial or legal skills. I worked with her and a local elder attorney to get the legal wills, power of attorney, medical power of attorney, etc., in place while my dad was still competent. I am not sure he understood all the details, but we got it done. I was committed to continue to help my mother in these areas, as she had enough to do taking care of my father. My wife supported my mother by being there whenever needed, driving my mother or father to doctor appointments, and doing homework on support groups/facilities, etc. It was a tough, but needed, duty for her.

My father had a good doctor, and when we told him our observations about Dad, without any significant testing, he concluded that it was dementia—likely the Alzheimer's type—and nothing medically could be done to relieve or stop it. Fortunately, we did not have a big problem convincing my father to give up driving. I think he knew. He was becoming more and more anxious and frustrated with what was happening to him. I still remember seeing him look at himself in the mirror and, almost in tears, saying, "I never thought I would get in this sad of shape." Perhaps he was remembering what happened to his older brother years before.

My wife took the lead in working with my mother to explore what support/resources were available to give her some relief. Most of the day-care programs were not appropriate for Dad since they were attended by folks who had progressed much further than he had. Consequently, his five-year journey with Alzheimer's took place at home with my mother.

One of the toughest decisions I had to make came in 1990. I was a D.C. native, my immediate and extended family was in the D.C.

area, and I had a great job with a major telecommunications company. However, my best friend from right after college had joined an entrepreneurial company in Boulder, CO in 1981. The company was growing very fast and he asked me to consider joining them. I was not looking for a change, but it was a great opportunity that I had to at least consider. After considering the pros and cons, talking with my mother (who was very supportive of my taking the opportunity), and talking with my wife who was also very supportive, I knew it was the right thing for me and my immediate family (we had a six-year-old daughter at the time).

BUT, could I abandon my father and mother and move to Boulder? So I sat down with them both. I am not sure Dad completely understood, but it was clear that he was not in favor of our moving. It was a tough one. I decided that I should do what was in the best interest of my immediate family and continue to support my parents the best I could. So we decided to move to Boulder. Travel between Denver and D.C. is pretty easy, so I committed to coming back to D.C. at least every four to six weeks to stay on top of my parents' affairs and spend time with them. I did that from May 1990 until November 1997, when my mother passed away.

After moving to Colorado in 1990, the travel to D.C. became easier because my job required me to be in Boston every other week. I was able to fly to D.C. from Boston and spend a day or two. While my mother was the primary caregiver, who was assisted by my wife — and after our move, by my sister-in-law — I took the lead on the financial and legal matters. That was easy compared to the day-to-day caregiving. However, the challenges took a toll on me as well.

My coping mechanisms fell into three areas: my job, running, and keeping a sense of humor. My job was very demanding, and keeping my energy focused there did not allow time to over-analyze and become preoccupied with the challenges of Alzheimer's. As a young adult, I had taken up running as a way to stay mentally and physically fit and it helped me a lot during this journey. I remember one time when I was in D.C., I told my mother that I was going on a forty-five minute run and she responded, "You don't really want to be here visiting." Ouch — but she was probably right and was venting some of the understandable frustration of dealing with Alzheimer's. It was on that run that I thought of my dad's certain death in the not-too-distant future and that, while very sad, he did not have any quality of life left and he would be in a better place after his death. That thought gave me some sense of peace during the remaining journey.

Lastly, keeping a sense of humor was important to me. Saying that, I always tried to be super-sensitive when I was around my dad. In the latter part of his journey, when I would try to review his financial situation with him (which was the best in his life), he just couldn't accept that he was in good financial shape. But even then, he would always express his appreciation of my help. It was frustrating for me as well, but my wife and I could joke about it when we were alone. An example of the humor was my Dad's inability to understand that he was in good financial shape and constantly insisting that, "We're getting low on money." When alone, my wife and I would declare "… we're getting low on money." As a depression era young adult, perhaps the long-term memory of "being low on money" was Dad's reality.

Our daughter was young during this five-year journey (three to eight years old). We certainly didn't try to shield her from my father, but we didn't try to explain it to her for two reasons: we thought she was too young to understand, and until the end, he always recognized us and was able to communicate reasonably. Perhaps we should have tried to give her an explanation, but I don't think it caused long-term negative issues. Today, at age thirty, she happily participates in many of the Alzheimer Association fund raising events that I am involved in.

By 1992, my father was getting worse, and my mother did get daytime in-home help. That helped give her some much needed relief, as my father required a lot of physical help. He knew who we were up until the end, but he was beginning to really suffer physically. He passed away on November 12, 1992 and the finality was sad, but also a relief. Having survived three years of war in Europe, Alzheimer's disease won the final battle. My mother lived another five years and passed away from heart issues. She was also a member of the Greatest Generation, who sacrificed in a much different way in the battle against Alzheimer's.

For the past several years, I have served on the Board of Directors of the Colorado Chapter Alzheimer's Association. It is a terrific organization and provides family support, classes, public awareness, and research for this dreaded disease. We are working very hard to make Alzheimer's a national priority. With baby boomers like me getting older, we are facing a huge problem if we don't find a cure. Alzheimer's is the sixth leading cause of death and the only one of the top ten killers that has no cure or effective treatment. If you need help or need information, please check the website at www.alz.org.

* * *

Dan Thomas *is Treasurer and Board member of the Alzheimer's Association (Colorado Chapter) and has served as Colorado Ambassador to United Sates Senators Mark Udall and Cory Gardner. Dan had a long career in the corporate finance world. Upon semi-retirement, he taught eight years in the business schools at CU and CSU and started serving as a volunteer in the non-profit world. He is a life member of the Virginia Jaycees, Past Board Chair of the People's Clinic in Boulder, Treasurer and Board member of Intercambio in Boulder, and is incoming Board Chair of Friendship Bridge. He enjoys hiking, snowshoeing, golf, and reading. Dan's family includes his wife Barbara and daughter Alison. For information about the Alzheimer's Association email:* info@alz.org.

15

Pray for Me

By Debra Wells

One day as John left the house for work at the usual 6:00 a.m., he said, "Pray for me." Several years earlier, his career had taken an intentional detour from the credit card business to education. As a public high school English teacher, he loved working with kids, teaching literature, and creating a fun learning environment. Recently, he was receiving a lot of attention about his performance from the school administration. He attributed their concerns to his hearing loss, for which he had worn hearing aids for several years.

I had seen indications of some type of issue with John's thought process for some time, but attributed his problems to stress. For several years, we had been the main caregivers for his parents, though they lived sixty-five miles from us in Colorado Springs. His mother died of cancer, and her decline was very difficult for him. Like most of our parents, she was fiercely independent. When disease weakened her to the point of not being able to care for herself or John's dad, she moved from a hospital stay to a care facility. She held John responsible for her situation and frequently lashed out at him. She died in December 2000, one month following the death of my father. Thirteen months later, John's father passed away in a nursing home close to our house. John visited him almost every day, even though his dad was suspicious and critical of him. Losing three parents in scarcely over a year was a stressful time for both of us.

Most caregivers of Alzheimer's patients look back at signs they should have noticed years earlier. This aberrant behavior gets excused and rationalized, and then suddenly it becomes apparent that something is very wrong. The eventual, ultimate attention-getter was an eleven-point performance improvement "corrective action" discipline memo that John's principal wrote. John was crestfallen—he'd been trying so hard to be a good teacher. I noticed he went over and over and over the homework he was "correcting" for the students. It seemed he could no longer put together the criteria for performance compared to the students' papers. He spent evenings and most of every weekend on schoolwork.

When John received previous directives to improve his work, I got involved. I helped him write lesson plans and came up with ideas for teaching. One of the books he taught was *To Kill a Mockingbird*. I found an interesting idea online about having students sketch out their idea of the layout of the town described by Harper Lee. I reviewed an example on the website and explained it to John. He seemed to think that it would be a good teaching tool. A few moments later, he asked me to explain it to him again, which I did. He went to the next room and began to work on the plan that would include this idea. He returned to where I was sitting, "Could you show me how that lesson with the map of the town would work again?" This went on for a few more rotations until we finally gave up on the idea.

It now seemed that it was time to seek help. Our doctor asked the right questions to get us directed toward appropriate diagnostic resources. (*Question*: Does John have difficulty with things he used to do well? *Answer*: He taught me how to use a computer; now he struggles with it.) The first step was an assessment of his current psychological state, in terms of depression. Six sessions led to the therapist's conclusion that John was depressed, but not to the extent that it would impact his cognitive skills. Concurrently, we pursued the potential physiological causes — brain tumor, stroke, and other neurological disorders. This is the one time that a positive result on these tests might not be the worst news. John's tests all came back negative.

The next month we got the "probable diagnosis" of Alzheimer's disease. The neuropsychological tests were the clincher — deficits in cognition could be clearly tracked to brain issues commonly associated with Alzheimer's disease. The doctor told us to get our affairs in order, while John could still participate in making decisions. He also told us to go to the Alzheimer's Association and learn as much as possible about the disease.

John and I cried a lot and began attending daily mass. He had always had a deep faith, and prayer was important to him. His routine included staying with a small group of parishioners to pray the rosary. Since I was still working, I had to get going to the other side of the city. John would then make the four to five mile trek back to our home on foot.

I should have noticed other indications of John's condition a year earlier. He was accepted into the formation of permanent deacons for the Archdiocese of Denver. The study for this involves the wives to a great extent. We would scale the foothills (in our car, of course) to reach Mother Cabrini Shrine, west of Denver. These regularly scheduled days would begin with a number of scriptural devotions found in the Roman Missal—Liturgy of the Hours. There is a multi-step process to locating the readings and prayers, which invariably confounded John. I was reluctant to seize the book from his hands to help him. How would that look to his "deacons-to-be" cohorts? Perhaps there were other deficits apparent to those who instructed him or administered the program. I know he wasn't socially interacting with the other candidates from our parish very effectively. John was asked—in a not-too-polite or dignity-maintaining manner—not to return for the continuation of his study for the diaconate. I felt a minor level of vindication when we revealed John's diagnosis to his former study partners.

In the early years of my conversion to Catholicism, Father Michael Walsh participated in healing masses. We attended a few of these with my mother during the last years of her life. She experienced some brief relief from her osteoporosis and emphysema.

Father Walsh had moved to a different parish and was doing healing masses on a regular basis. News accounts described his gift. John and I attended one such mass on September 12, 2002, two months after his diagnosis. We arrived fairly early, about thirty minutes before the start of mass, and sat halfway back on the left side of the sanctuary. The pews began to fill with a diverse group. Some people held rosary beads, and some had Bibles. Others seemed to be new to a Catholic church (the healing, Father would explain, is open to all). It was apparent that those in attendance had a variety of physical impairments. Some had hair loss from their treatments; others limped or had splints supporting injured limbs.

The full mass was celebrated, with an especially meaningful homily about forgiveness. Father tied the ability to physically heal to the ability to heal from other, non-physical wounds through the power of forgiveness. Father called for testimony from those in attendance who had previously been healed. One woman described her lack of Multiple Sclerosis symptoms after experiencing the healing. Another woman related a story of having leukemia cured. There were accounts of hearing being restored and an end to debilitating headaches.

We observed that two strapping men had placed themselves near those receiving the healing sacrament from Father. As the recipients went through the healing process, some briefly lost consciousness. The fit young men were there to help guide the person to the floor, where he or she usually recovered within a few minutes, stood up, and returned to sit in a pew.

I accompanied John to the altar when his turn came, and we approached Father Walsh. After hearing John's diagnosis and request for healing (and registering some amount of shock, as he'd known John from his prior parish), Father stated that I should also receive the sacrament. Father Walsh's experienced healing hands administered the oils to John's forehead and palms. John fell backwards, and the two men guided him gently to the floor, where he remained for about fifteen minutes.

"I tried to fight it!" he said in a groggy voice. Back in the pew, John was clearly moved, but appeared relaxed and happy. Later he would recount the experience of being overtaken by a wash of golden light. He said he thought his "brain connections" were being repaired during this time. Father recommended that we read certain passages of scripture aloud daily — which we did — to continue the healing.

A few days after the service, John announced he was healed and would no longer be taking his medications. I immediately protested, "Honey, who knows how this healing works?! Maybe that's the fulfillment of the promise of healing. They have all these new drugs coming on the market. Maybe you're taking a new unique combination of supplements and drugs that will be very effective. It's important that you continue to take your medications!"

Immediately I thought of a story that I've heard embedded in at least a few homilies: A person is stranded during a flood and prays to God for help. He is sure that God will answer his pleas. As the water rises steadily, a neighbor comes by in a boat and offers a way out. The stranded person rejects the offer, "No thank you - God is going to rescue me." A number of other conveyances appear on the scene, all of which the stranded person refuses. When the person perishes in the flood, he is greeted at the pearly gates by God. "Why didn't you save me?" asks the victim, to which God replies, "Well, I sent a boat, a raft, a canoe…what did you want?!" "John," I said, after telling him this story again, "Don't turn down the boat!"

John's assertion was that his healing was a gift from God and by taking the drugs he was doubting the healing. I convinced him to call Father Walsh to discuss it. As I anticipated, Father Walsh supported my advice to John.

As the years went by, John's condition was more stable than I had anticipated. At our "younger onset" couples support group I felt like a bragger. "John still reads. John takes walks on his own. John can write checks (but not balance the checkbook). John watches PBS programs during the day and tells me all about them when I get home in the evening." Yet, John was mighty confused at times. He couldn't operate the stove or microwave (and thankfully, didn't try). He couldn't adjust the thermostat or attach the dog's harness. The calendar had become a mystery to him. He wouldn't be able to handle most household emergencies.

We had heard that the experience of most younger-onset sufferers was that the progression was more accelerated; a decline to full-time care would probably be only a few years away. We thank God that our experience was almost the opposite for several years. I think, perhaps, that when John felt the golden light wash over him, the destructive force of his degenerative illness was slowed down.

Although I'm not usually the first one to jump up and make a speech, I felt compelled to deliver a testimony of our story at a healing mass about a year after John's experience. I was fairly brief, but I contrasted some of John's symptoms that led to the diagnosis with positive changes I'd noted since the addition of a (then only available in Europe) medication memantine (now available in the U.S. under the brand name Namenda®). John was now able to follow a complete baseball game and tell me the inning-by-inning account later in the day.

I concluded that God's healing power is a mystery. We were very thankful that we had this additional time together. John passed away in 2014. I reflect on this healing session as one of the major positive events of his illness.

People ask me how I coped with all that happened, all that was demanded of me in providing care for John while I worked full-time outside the home. I had help in many different areas. We brought in professional caregiver/companions fairly early in his illness to take John out a few days a month. This gave him a chance to experience the world a bit, independent of me. We also had a cleaning service that came in every few weeks. Our cleaning person was wonderful with John and our dog, Murphy, and provided companionship in between her mopping and vacuuming.

The support groups John and I were part of were an important outlet for both of us. I actually attended two groups — one couples group with John, and one just for caregivers. Having the opportunity to express frustrations and fears and to talk about setbacks, disappointments, and occasional joys made a major difference. Throughout my experience, I'd think about the way I expressed my thoughts about some aspect of the progression of the disease to the group. Whether it was John losing the remote to the TV set just days after we purchased it, or dealing with major losses in terms of abilities, I knew that I would have a friendly, understanding interaction with a knowledgeable person who had already been down this path or was now on the journey, like me.

I think of John dozens of times a day, and find myself smiling about jokes he made or a nice experience we shared. The time I remember him most vividly, and almost feel him by my side, is when I attend mass. It's an honor to be able to heed his request, "pray for me."

* * *

Deb Wells *became involved in the activities of the Alzheimer's Association during her husband's illness. After her caregiving duties concluded, she continued her role on the public policy committee, facilitating a support group, interacting with Federal elected officials, and speaking at education seminars for the Association. In late 2015 she accepted an opportunity to join the staff of the Colorado Chapter in the role of Vol-*

unteer and Statistics Coordinator. She can be reached at <u>debkwells@</u> <u>comcast.net</u>. *Deb enjoys traveling with friends, and spending time with her dog, Buddy, in the home she and John shared.*

Part Three

✕

Healing Modalities

16

Acupuncture

Acupuncture is a form of Chinese medicine that has been practiced for thousands of years. It is based on the theory that energy, or chi, flows through your body along pathways called meridians. Two acupuncturists share how they use acupuncture to help reduce stress and improve quality of life for caregivers and people with dementia.

"Energy flows where intention goes." – Author unknown

Classical Five Element Acupuncture

By Dr. **Jim Brooks**, MD

I have been a practicing psychiatrist for the past thirty-three years. My practice is eclectic. I treat with a combination of allopathic psychopharmacology, herbal and nutritional medicines, psycho-therapy, and Classical Five Element Acupuncture (CFEA). As a general psychiatrist, I treat adults and children, and address all psychiatric disorders, including anxiety disorders, PTSD, depression, schizophrenia, bipolar disorder, ADHD, Autism Spectrum Disorders, and Dementia.

Having treated thousands of patients over the years, my preference is to use more natural methods of treatment, rather than allopathic medicine, whenever possible. This is because of the side effects—some of them quite serious—that occur with allopathic treatment. The higher degree of side effects, in my opinion, is due to the fact that allopathic medicines are synthetically made ("man made"). Because the drugs are synthetic, the human body typically does not recognize these chemicals because they appear foreign to the body. Also, the dosage of these compounds is often very potent. Hence, side effects commonly occur, either due to the body's natural immune reaction to these compounds, or due to the direct toxic effect they can produce.

Herbal medicines, on the other hand, when used with proper knowledge and training, typically are prepared in combination with other herbal preparations, which has the overall effect of mitigating side effects. Natural herbs, properly and safely prepared, are seen as "friendly" substances by the body's immune system, and also the dosing is more compatible with human physiology, so that the body doesn't react negatively against these natural preparations.

For the past fourteen years, I have been using Classical Five Element Acupuncture to treat anxiety, acute and chronic stress, depression, fatigue, chronic pain, and neurological and cognitive disorders. This system of acupuncture is holistic, which makes it particularly effective. Through pulse diagnosis, the practitioner can assess specific blocks in the flow of life energy, which is also known as chi or prana. Through simple application of a few needles, these blocks can be completely removed. Because the chi energy flow is seen in Chinese medicine as critical to healthy functioning of the mind, body, and spirit, when this energy becomes blocked (kind of like water gets blocked when the hose gets kinked up), imbalances and, ultimately, diseases begin to develop.

Another unique and important feature of Classical Five Element Acupuncture is that a properly trained practitioner can detect which of the five elements (fire, earth, metal, water, and wood) is fundamentally imbalanced in anyone. According to Chinese medicine, imbalance and disease are a direct result of imbalances in these five elements. This diagnosis is made through sensing imbalanced color, sound, odor, and emotion (CSOE). Each of the elements has a characteristic imbalanced CSOE, and when the practitioner makes the diagnosis, he or she can pick appropriate points to restore elemental balance in the patient. In this way, Classical Five Element Acupuncture is a wonderful and very powerful and effective natural method for preventing and treating illness.

What I love about practicing this system of Chinese medicine is that there are virtually no side effects. This system is unique because, although it helps a person's symptoms, it is not symptom focused. Rather, it triggers the body's own natural immunity and ability to self-repair, and enhances functioning of mind, body, and spirit. Many people ask, "Do the needles hurt?" Sometimes you might experience a "dull ache" that quickly dissipates. The good news is that the occasional slight discomfort is significantly outweighed by the overall benefits from the treatment.

Typically, the "rule of thumb" is that recovery from any health problem with effective systems of natural medicine takes about one quarter to one half the time the condition has been present. So, if the condition has lasted four years, then it may take about one to two years of treatment to fully recover. However, this is only a guide rule. I have seen many medical/psychiatric conditions clear up very quickly—in a matter of weeks or months—regardless of how long they have previously been present. To be fair, however, there are some severe conditions that may need on-going treatment, and even may need to be supplemented with allopathic and other methodologies of treatment. In my experience, a person will often start feeling some relief from symptoms very soon after starting treatment. With chronic stress related to long-term caregiving, and most other health issues, regular treatment is recommended every 1-4 weeks, depending on the nature of the problem, and its severity, acuity and chronicity.

One of my patients has advanced Alzheimer's disease. Her caregiver, whom I'll call Mary, has been a long-term partner. Mary gets very stressed, frustrated, and fatigued at times, due to the relentless sacrifices she has had to make. There are moments of tenderness and joy in her role as caregiver, but her caregiving efforts have resulted in health issues of her own, brought about by chronic stress.

About one and a half years ago, Mary decided to get Classical Five Element treatment for herself, to better cope with the chronic stress. After each treatment, she feels a boost in spirit, and a renewed sense of well-being, hope, courage, and energy. She comes in for treatment every few weeks, and is very careful not to miss her regular sessions, as they give her the stamina she needs to continue in her role as primary caregiver.

CFEA can be helpful to individuals with dementia. It can have very powerful effects on enhancing the brain functioning. Studies on acupuncture have shown that it can enhance neuroendocrine functioning and blood flow to the brain. Practically speaking, I have seen symptomatic improvements in memory, alertness, anxiety, agitation, aggression, irritability, and depression. In most cases, dementia patients tolerate the treatments quite well, especially with the support and encouragement of their caregivers. Obviously, due to the chronicity of most forms of dementia, weekly or bi-weekly ongoing treatment is ideal.

* * *

Jim Brooks, MD, has been practicing psychiatry in Fairfield, Iowa for the last thirty-two years. He also is a Classical Five Element Acupuncturist, an Ayurvedic physician, and a practitioner of Zero Balancing. He is the author of many book chapters on the application of natural medicine to the field of Psychiatry, and he is the co-author of the book Ayurvedic Secrets To Longevity *and* Total Health *(Prentice Hall publishing). He can be reached on his website,* AdventuresInPartnering.com, *and by phone, 541-469-6097.*

Utmost Source

By **Sarah Brooks**

In Chinese medicine the heart is called the supreme controller, the "designated leader of all the other officials." When the supreme controller in a person is sick, the person can experience sadness and abandonment. Fear can prevail. From this place, all kinds of dis-ease can arise. When Natural Law is restored in a person, love, warmth, and the divine connection that reminds us we are not alone helps heal the dis-ease. It is vital for health. (Adapted from *Janerit of the Points: A Work in Progress,* J.B. Worsley and J.R. Worlsey.)

When Jane became sick, her mind and body declined quickly. She was once a woman in our spiritual community with a high-powered job and was respected by many. Some considered her to be famous for her accomplishments. Her physical and mental decline was a shock to everyone. Her life-partner, Tom, tried for months to care for her at home as best he could, which soon became impossible when Jane became unable to take care of herself. As an acupuncturist, I was called to treat Jane about four months after she was transferred to the local nursing home.

The nursing home stank, and people screamed, "You are the crazy ones! Let me outta here," when anyone walked through the doors. Jane was in the locked ward and having health complications such as bladder infections, nail infections, and flu. She was also having paranoid thoughts, her body was very rigid, and she seemed fearful all the time.

Jane had to be wheeled into my office for her first treatment. Her body was so tense, it was like one giant cramped muscle. Her hands were tight claws, her ankles hardly moved, her face was cramped, and her eyes looked dull. She was having trouble adjusting to the nursing home. She got angry and constantly talked about killing people or people who were trying to kill her. She fought the staff by becoming rigid and non-compliant for simple things like going to eat with the others or getting out of bed. She even fell and hit her head one time. She also experienced chronic urinary tract infections (UTIs) and was susceptible to colds and other viruses. Her eyes would get crusty and her toenails had a chronic pussy fungus.

I had worked with cancer patients going through chemotherapy, people who had lost all hope to live, or who experienced chronic back pain. But after practicing as an acupuncturist only three years at the time, I realized that she was the sickest person I had seen, in terms of chronic illness. Jane couldn't even tell anyone sensibly what was wrong. It was hard to find (needle) points for her based on the interpretations from her doctors, nurses, and Tom. I have to admit, I really wondered at the time if the acupuncture would produce any positive effects in this woman.

It took about two to three months of weekly treatments to begin seeing the dramatic changes from the acupuncture. At the end of that year, Judy Worsley, my master teacher of Classical Five Element Acupuncture, came to town to do consultations for many of my patients, as she does once a year. I really wanted her advice for treating Jane. Judy and I traveled to the memory care home one late afternoon after seeing patients all day at my office. Judy diagnosed Jane and refined the treatments I had been giving her. From that point on, Jane really began to take off. It didn't take long before her urinary tract infections went away. I treated her every week for a year and those infections have never come back. Her cognition improved a bit. She had already calmed down a lot from the regular treatments, but she started emanating pure bliss. Now all the staff comments regularly on what a complete joy it is to be around her.

At first I admit feeling sympathy for Jane's friends and co-workers, who still refuse to visit her in her new home. But I adjusted as I got more comfortable with the staff, and Jane's room is quiet and cozy. Even when the other patients sometimes try to come in during her treatments, Jane just sits back in her chair and laughs, and so I laugh too. Tom, her devoted life partner, decorated the room with lots of family photos, free standing lamps, and framed pictures of her beloved guru. She also has a radio and a TV with a DVD player, so Tom sometimes brings in romantic comedies or documentaries for them to watch together.

Jane cries tears through her smile when she sees Tom walk in the door. He continues to bring her organic foods and supplements and to read her his original poetry. Since Jane's love and warmth has been restored, I don't even see her as a sick person, because she is glowing from the inside out. When I go to her room now, I think of it as her own private cave where she is retired and genuinely content. It is away from the noise of cell phones and national news about random shootings. Although Jane barely talks anymore, the people who visit her say she radiates light, and the comments she does make seem to be just right for the moment.

Compassion has kept me steadfast, and Tom has been a great influence on me. He shows so much loyalty towards Jane, caring for her and talking sweetly to her, even when she is in a negative or obsessive mood. He accompanies her to every appointment, manages everything from her finances to her herbs and supplements, and sees to her receiving acupuncture and massage therapy. He brings organic veggies to the care facility for them to cook for her so she gets proper nutrition.

I continue to give Jane follow-up acupuncture treatments at her care facility instead of at my office. It is not the ideal situation for me as a practitioner because I cannot control the nursing home environment as I do in my office. I would like to treat her on a table, which allows me to move her around more easily and reach her back readily. I treat her in a reclining chair in her room, which makes treating her more difficult. However, Tom helps me with this.

I recently saved a message on my phone from Tom when he visited Jane after one of her acupuncture treatments. Tom called to thank me for the treatment and Jane was in the background laughing away. I thought it was such a sweet message from the two of them. That day Jane was in her chair when I first came into the room, and she was resting quietly as usual with her eyes closed. She had a contented look on her face. Her eyes were soft and her lips were closed. She had just woken from a nap and the staff helped her into her recliner. She had her neck brace on, as she tends to hold her head rigidly to the left. The physical rigidity in her body is something we continually work on.

I asked her how she was doing that day, and she replied, "Goooood," in a long, sweet voice. Then she began to ramble on in words and sentences I could not recognize, as she often does. It's as though she knows what she is saying, but she is talking so fast we cannot understand her. Sometimes she will slow down and either ask me a question or answer a question I've asked her. Towards the end of the treatment that day she asked, "What does this one do?" I told her it was relaxing her body and her mind. The fact that she asked that after two years of treatment and very little coherent speech was incredible to me. I asked her if she wanted to move to a different facility, because this was a current topic for her. She replied simply, "I'm fine." It was heartwarming to hear her make these remarks.

Over the last two years, I have seen Jane change in incredible ways. She has become not only pleasant to be around, but a downright light-being, shining and smiling, laughing and giggling. Her immunity has been strengthened, and she doesn't get sick when others in the facility do. She no longer has the infections in her nails or bladder or gets flu symptoms. In fact, she has not been sick with ANYTHING viral or bacterial since she first started her acupuncture treatments. She no longer panics like she used to, and doesn't talk incoherently about things that scare her. There are good and bad days, however, just as we all have. But Jane's reactions are, more or less, within a normal range of experience for someone with advanced dementia. It seems as if she has accepted her condition, but have we?

Sometimes Jane is beaming with joy when I first walk in the room, and she smiles and comments on how beautiful I am. I kiss her forehead and we both gaze lovingly into each other's eyes. The connections I have made with this woman have really changed my life, and it is impossible for me to see her as a "sick" person. I can see that the divine connection in Jane has been restored, as she radiates warmth, compassion, and contentment from inside herself. She doesn't seem lonely, scared, or in physical dis-ease as many of the other patients in her unit are. Even though her speech and physical body don't look the way a normal person's would, I believe she is living in a quiet place within herself, based on the warmth and humor she radiates to those who are around her.

The heart has a direct relationship with divine presence, and when the natural order is restored here, a person's body, mind, and spirit are in a stable state knowing there is a supreme order. (Adapted from *Janerit of the Points: A Work in Progress,* J.B. Worsley and J.R. Worlsey.) And this, I believe, Jane has in abundance.

* * *

Sarah Brooks MA, Lic. Ac., received her Masters of Acupuncture from Colorado's Institute of Taoist Education and Acupuncture in early 2008. She formerly conducted research at Dana-Farber Cancer Institute and Harvard Medical School. Sarah is certified to practice acupuncture by the Iowa Board of Medicine and the National Certification Commission for Acupuncture and Oriental Medicine. She has a thriving acupuncture practice in Fairfield, Iowa. Reach her at: <u>classicalacupuncture@hotmail. com</u> *and* <u>iowafiveelement.com</u>.

17

Animal-Assisted Therapy

*W*arm *puppies definitely create happiness, and in this chapter you'll learn about the joys and rewards that result from playing with and touching animals. Discover various methods, benefits, and cautions of Animal-Assisted Therapy. Included are safe ways that family members can engage with an animal to diffuse highly charged emotional situations.*

"Animals are such agreeable friends – they ask no questions; they pass no criticisms." – George Eliot

By **Diana McQuarrie**

Animal-Assisted Therapy (AAT) is recognized by the National Institute of Mental Health as a type of psychotherapy for treating depression and other mood disorders. Spending time with an animal seems to promote a sense of emotional connectedness and well-being. Touching and playing with animals is a wonderful way for families coping with Alzheimer's disease to experience joy, fun, and laughter.

Animal-Assisted Therapy is gaining popularity as part of therapy programs in memory care facilities. Memory impaired patients often withdraw from people and find animal interaction easier and non-threatening. Other patients simply enjoy the physical contact with an animal. Just being in the presence of a dog can uplift or sooth some people. When people interact with pets, the physiological response is a lowering of blood pressure and an increase in the neurochemicals associated with relaxation and bonding. These effects can help ameliorate behavioral and psychological symptoms of dementia.

Several small studies suggest that the presence of a dog reduces aggression and agitation, and promotes social behavior in people with dementia. One study showed that having aquariums in the dining rooms of memory care homes stimulates residents to eat more and to maintain a healthier weight. When a dog is brought to visit memory impaired individuals (either at home or a facility), unexpected and positive reactions occur. Some patients who have refused to speak will talk to the dog, and others who have refused to move might pet the dog.

My daughter often brought her Miniature Schnauzer, Paco, to the home where Morris lived. Paco always brightened the day for Morris and the other residents. Paco would run around scrounging for crumbs and sniffing the residents' feet. Some residents reached out to touch him. One lady liked to hold him like a baby. She'd place a napkin on his head, pretending it was a hat. Paco created a bit of a stir, but he brought a smile to everyone's face, including mine.

The human-animal bond goes beyond the mind and is centered in the heart. It can nurture us in ways that nothing else can. Sometimes a person with memory loss won't be able to recognize a spouse, but can recognize a beloved pet. Just three days before Morris died, a friend visited him with his trained pet therapy dog. Morris was bedridden, dehydrated, and non-communicative, but he opened his eyes and reached out for the dog.

If your loved one is used to being around animals, has had a pet, or if there is an animal that he or she is familiar with, by all means encourage the interaction to continue. It's an easy, wonderful way to promote ease and happiness among care partners. If there is no family pet, consider Animal-Assisted Therapy, which is facilitated by a professional therapist and carried out by a trained team. Diana McQuarrie, MSOL, founder and executive director emeritus of Denver Pet Partners, has been working in the field of Animal-Assisted Therapy for almost two decades and has extensive experience incorporating therapy animals as a treatment modality with Alzheimer's patients and their caregivers. She relays her professional experience.

Interview with Diana McQuarrie

Animal-Assisted Therapy incorporates a skilled handler-animal team in goal directed intervention as an integral part of the treatment process. The therapy animals and their handlers who work in this field are screened to meet certain criterion and go through a training and assessment. The team collaborates with a credentialed therapist to determine the appropriate therapy animal interaction to complement treatment goals. During the course of treatment, the team is guided by a health care professional, who measures and evaluates the progress made by the patient. Since AAT is becoming more of a mainstream treatment modality, it is reimbursable by some insurance companies, just as other types of therapy.

Animal-Assisted activities do not have to always be guided by therapists who bill for their services. Often, a trained handler will bring his or her therapy dog for a "meet and greet" situation where the goal-directed activities are meant to improve quality of life through the interaction. Also, pet owners who go through the training with their dogs volunteer their time to try to alleviate stress, depression, and anxiety for diverse populations, including the elderly, dementia patients, and hospitalized children.

There are a lot of things to consider when incorporating AAT with individuals who have dementia or Alzheimer's disease. First of all, when we're setting up a treatment plan for a patient with Alzheimer's, we have to consider the stage of the disease that the patient is in. Clearly there are different techniques used for each stage.

If the person is in the earlier stages of Alzheimer's, we strive to work towards a goal to increase their ability to engage, to help them reminisce, and to brighten their mood. If we want to improve socialization and communication for that individual, we encourage the patient to engage with the animal by brushing it, giving it commands, and trying to teach it something new. This draws the person out and helps improve his or her general social interaction.

This was scientifically demonstrated in 2002 and 2003 studies that were published in the *American Journal of Alzheimer's Disease and Other Dementias*. The nine-week pilot study was conducted in 2003 in two New England nursing homes that offered therapeutic recreation programs. Each intervention group in the pilot study consisted of therapeutic recreation staff members, therapy dog(s), and the therapy dog handler(s). The studies found that the agitated behaviors of the participants decreased immediately following the intervention phase and increased during the follow-up phase of the study.

Another treatment goal of AAT is to reduce loneliness and isolation. Some of the techniques we incorporate for this includes having patients reminisce about the past while they interact with the dog. We encourage direct eye contact and ask questions to promote conversation, such as "Have you ever had a dog? What was its name? Was it a male or female? Did you go on walks with it?" Interaction with a therapy dog can trigger memories in people with long-term memory loss.

For patients that are in the early and moderate stages of Alzheimer's, we might set up an agility course for the patient and the therapy dog to walk through. The patient can have the choice to become proactively involved by helping set up the course. The exercise is cognitively stimulating and becomes an empowering cooperative plan that helps the patient express feelings and accomplish something with the handler and the animal. The patient also engages in conversation with the handler and dog, and receives appropriate affection from the dog. These experiences help improve the patients' overall social functioning.

We work both one-on-one with patients and in groups with a therapist present. If we're working in a group setting, the whole room lights up when a handler-animal team walks in. The handler introduces the dog to the group, and may talk about the breed or how it needs to be groomed. The care and attention required to maintain the dog's health is used as a transference for the patients to relate to what is required in their own lives to sustain health and well-being. Staff members and other visitors may come in, and regardless of each person's situation, there is a common thread. Everyone is focused on engaging with the therapy animal. It's comparable to what music does for people. It doesn't matter what is going on in your life, nearly everyone can relate to the universal language of music. Likewise with an animal, unless there is a phobia or prior negative experiences with an animal, most people enjoy the interaction and benefit from it.

Group work draws people out, and they can talk back and forth and share information and stories about the animal. Patients in the earlier stages of Alzheimer's will remember the animals' names and that the animals were there the previous week. They start to get to know the handler and the dog. It stimulates their memory and it triggers past experiences for them, which they sometimes like to share with other members of the group.

If the patient brushes the dog, helps walk the dog, or makes eye contact with the dog, it is stimulating to both the patient and the dog. The patient receives positive feedback from the animal and both receive affection. This helps to brighten the patient's affect and mood, and is especially effective when working with people who are depressed. The interaction takes their mind off things that are creating anxiety for them, such as having to go to a doctor's appointment or take medication twice a day. Or the interaction is simply a relief from the symptoms of Alzheimer's disease. The bonus for caregivers who might be observing all this is that the scenario produces a calming influence and relieves their anxiety, as well.

Some of the other treatment goals aim at improving memory and recall, which is significant when working with people with Alzheimer's. When we regularly visit a patient who starts to reminisce, we can continue on that line of discussion and ask questions about the animal. If the person recalls things about the animal's care, we will repeat information about the animal on subsequent visits. Then we might ask the patient to repeat information about the breed of dog and ask questions such as "Has the dog been here to visit you before? How do you think the animal is feeling now?" It encourages patients to think about something beyond their own world.

This all depends on the patient's cognitive abilities, of course. And we work only with people who have no phobia of animals. As the patient's cognitive ability declines, the techniques we use change. Working with patients with Alzheimer's is always somewhat unpredictable, depending upon the person's mood, physical condition, and the environment. We wouldn't be working with a patient who is severely agitated or could pose a danger to the animal and/or handler. We would never go into a secured unit and dress a therapy dog in a costume, for example. We can't anticipate the triggers. We always consider what is best for the patients, based on where they are cognitively. In its pure form, AAT is a very effective treatment modality if it's done safely with trained professionals and/or volunteers, together with the appropriate therapy animal and with a plan to achieve specific outcomes.

On one occasion, my therapy dog and I were working with patients in a secured dementia facility. A lady with Alzheimer's approached us; all dressed up with her coat and purse and ready to go somewhere. She came up to me and said, "Can you let me know when you're leaving? I'm going to go out with you because my son is picking me up." Of course I knew better than to let her out of the unit, and I let the staff know about her request. An aide told me, "She does that every day. She gets dressed and waits for her son to pick her up. But he doesn't even live around here and isn't scheduled to come."

As a therapy animal handler, it's sad to see these types of situations. You look into those people's eyes, and wish you could bring back their memory and heal everything that's happening in their brain. I spent time with that lady on a weekly basis. I don't know if she remembered me from week to week, but she always remembered my therapy dog and eagerly interacted with both of us. She'd perk up and talk about her son, which she did not do with the staff. The dog was a huge impetus for her to engage in conversation. It was a real milestone.

Another time, I was working on a weekly basis in an assisted living center with individuals who had moderate cognitive decline. These people would remember that I came every week and that my dog's name was Shana. When I arrived, they would light up with clear recognition. They brushed Shana, and this led them to talking and reminiscing about their animals. Although they didn't have much short-term memory, they were able to talk about their childhood and what it was like growing up. It really benefited them to reminisce. It was fabulous.

Loneliness can be easier to endure in the company of animals. Many of the patients we work with are very lonely. Their spouses may have passed away and their families don't always live in the same city, so visits are infrequent and meaningful personal interaction is limited. Afterwards I always spoke with the staff who told me that it was amazing how I was able to draw these people out. Otherwise, they'd just be sitting here not doing anything, they said. All of these visits and experiences were equally rewarding for me, regardless of the stage of Alzheimer's these patients were in. While Animal-Assisted Therapy is a team effort, the credit for being able to draw these people out belongs mostly to my therapy dog.

Touch is one of the last of the five senses to go. We've worked in hospice with patients with Alzheimer's in end-of-life situations. When patients place their hands on a dog wonderful tactile experience as evidenced by their response. Their face might soften, or they might smile. It's always amazing to witness that. I'm convinced it's from the connection they feel with the animal.

Animal-Assisted Therapy, done according to standards of practice and with strict adherence to risk management and safety, with all the training and on-going education it demands, is hard work but very rewarding. The power of the human animal bond to promote healing and enhance lives is extraordinary.

* * *

Diana McQuarrie is the Founder and Executive Director Emeritus of Denver Pet Partners, one of the largest Pet Partner Affiliates in the nation, and the owner of Altus AAT Solutions, providing professional consulting and instruction in the effective delivery of human-animal interaction services in the healthcare, education, and child welfare fields. Diana has developed international curricula and taught volunteers and healthcare professionals how to integrate animals as part of the therapeutic treatment team.Contact: dianam@altussolutions.org.

For more information on Denver Pet Partners, Animal-Assisted Therapy, and how you can become a volunteer, visit www.denverpetpartners.org/index.html or email info@denverpetpartners.org.

* * *

Interview with Heidi Zeller-Dart

I registered Guinness and myself as a pet partner team with the American Humane Association. Guinness is a full-bred black Lab and was one year old when we started doing visits to memory care homes and nursing homes. He's very smart and sensitive, and picks up on clients' emotions and triggers reactions, which makes him a good therapy dog. When we are at a facility, he knows he is at work and that he needs to be obedient. He does a good job most of the time.

I worked with one client at Juniper Village memory care home for more than a year. We'd go every week for an hour or so, and even though we went to visit one particular person, we ended up spending time with many residents. No one knew my name, but Guinness wore a blue badge and everyone knew his name. He was the light that caught everyone's eye and drew everyone in. People were drawn to him, and he would trigger memories for everyone.

One thing he did was to bring people together. Sometimes I'd walk into Juniper Village and the residents would be sleeping in chairs or in their rooms. There usually wasn't much social interaction going on. Guinness would come in and the people would start talking to each other. I'd carry around a photo album of him as a puppy, swimming, or taking a bath. That would open up conversation, and even people who weren't verbal would start talking.

Guinness particularly liked my client's room. The lighting was dim and sometimes she'd just sit there and not move, and he'd be content just lying on her feet. She was a loving, affectionate person and she'd reach out to touch him. She enjoyed the physical connection she had with him. Guinness made her smile and she'd talk non-stop, even though I was unable to understand most of what she said. When it was time to leave, Guinness was stubborn. I'd have to pull him out of the room because he didn't want to leave.

Sometimes our client was in a group activity, and Guinness and I would walk around and people would reach out to pet him or feed him treats. I'd feel bad because everyone was paying attention to Guinness instead of listening to the person leading the activity. But having Guinness there brought people together. He helped create a setting for some people to get out of their boring routine of being alone. A warm, soft, friendly animal elicits a reaction. I'd bring a couple of brushes so people could brush Guinness. It's a soothing activity and it helps people feel that they are caring for something. Guinness also helped the staff feel relaxed and happy, which supports them in their care of the patients.

Comforting the Dying

The first time Guinness and I went to spend time with someone who was dying was at the request of the family. The patient was a dog lover. I'm not even sure the person was conscious, but I told her that we were there. I described Guinness for her and told her about him and she did touch him. The second time we went to assist a family with a dying relative, Guinness and I spent time with the patient's young granddaughter and her mom. That was comforting for the family to focus on and laugh with Guinness. Our presence helped sooth and relax them.

I've been doing basic office therapy a few years, and I plan to incorporate AAT in my private practice. Last year I started doing equine psychotherapy. We have a farm in Berthoud, Colorado where I'll be creating an Animal-Assisted Therapy program with horses, chickens, pigs, dogs, and cats, to start. Guinness will definitely be a part of that.

* * *

Since graduating with a Master's Degree from the University of Denver's Counseling Psychology Program in 2009, **Heidi Zeller-Dart** *MA, LPC has been in private practice working with individuals experiencing grief/ loss, mood disorders, interpersonal challenges, and PTSD stemming from childhood trauma. Heidi has a deep appreciation for the healing power of the human-animal bond. Email Heidi at:* heidi.c.zeller@gmail.com.

* * *

References

Filan, Susan L. and Robert H. Llewellyn-Jones. 2006. "Animal-assisted therapy for dementia: a review of the literature." *International Psychogeriatrics.* 18(4): 597-608.

Richeson, Nancy E. 2003. "Effects of animal-assisted therapy on agitated behaviors and social interactions of older adults with dementia." *American Journal of Alzheimer's Disease and Other Dementias.* 18(6): 353-358.

Tribet J, Boucharlat M, Myslinski M. 2008. "[Animal-assisted therapy for people suffering from severe dementia]." (article in French). *L Encéphale*. 34(2):183-6.

18

Aromatherapy

Aside from providing a pleasant scent, specific odors can evoke memories and even change our moods. Learn about the wonderful science of aromatherapy, how specific oils can reduce stress and depression, and how you can blend oils to use in a diffuser or in a lotion for daily use for yourself and your loved one.

"The way to health is to have an aromatic bath
and scented massage every day." – Hippocrates

By **Laraine Pounds**, RN MSN BSN, CMT

Aromatherapy can be a resource of comfort to you and your care partner by providing an easy, natural way to reduce stress and anxiety and uplift mood. *Aromatherapy* refers to the inhalation and topical application of essential oils obtained from aromatic plant material to maintain health and well-being, and to restore imbalances on the physical, emotional, mental, and spiritual levels.

Essential Oils are distilled, highly concentrated extracts from whole plants and from various parts of the plant, including the flowers, leaves, fruit, rind, wood, berries, roots, and resin. These aromatic oils can be used individually or blended together for various uses. Essential oils are easy to use, affordable, and versatile for personal self-care and the care of others. They can be added to body lotion, massage oil, or used by inhalation from a spritz or diffuser, personal inhaler, or directly from the bottle.

Many health food stores sell essential oils and have tester bottles on display, making it easy and fun to sample the various fragrances to identify personal preferences. This could be an enjoyable activity with your care partner, in early stages of decline, who is still able to discern and communicate personal aromatic preferences. Many essential oil companies offer pre-blended synergy oils for specific use, such as boosting the immune system, relaxation and sleep, or for uplifting and invigorating purposes.

To ensure you are buying a pure essential oil and not synthetic fragrance oil, look for the botanical name of the plant and the phrase "pure essential oil" on the label. Generally, "nature identical" synthetic fragrance oils or fragrance blends are not used in traditional aromatherapy; however, if someone enjoys a fragrance such as gardenia, lilac, or frangipani that is only available in a synthetic fragrance blend, there is nothing wrong with using such a fragrance for aromatic pleasure.

History

Healers in every major culture, including ancient Egypt, China, and India, have utilized scented ointments and oils for healing and for their spiritual and psycho-emotional effects. Many religious traditions enjoyed incense, using cedar, cypress, sandalwood, and spices such as cinnamon. Before distillation evolved, fragrance oils were obtained through expression, maceration, and infusion in a vegetable oil. Queen Cleopatra is well known for her appreciation of aromatics and reportedly used roses, jasmine, frankincense, and juniper berry in bathing, cosmetics, religious rituals, and perfumery.

Early Christians held fragrance in high regard and embraced the symbolism of plant aroma representing the soul of the plant. Mary Magdalene anointed Christ with healing oils infused with spikenard, rose, marjoram, frankincense, and myrrh. In the first century AD, Dioscorides, a Greek physician, documented the properties of many of the herbs and aromatics that we use today as essential oils, including cypress, myrrh, frankincense, juniper, pine, rosemary, cardamom, basil, fennel, rose, and thyme.

Many monasteries in the Middle Ages grew herbal gardens and were noted for plant therapies. Hildegard of Bingen, a Benedictine nun, studied, practiced, and wrote about plant medicine. She used lavender for a variety of purposes and wrote about the connection between the body, emotions, and spirit and role of hope, joy, and affection for a strong immune system.

Florence Nightingale described creating pleasing environments for healing and documented her uses of rose and myrrh during the Crimean War. Rene Gattefosse, a French chemist, coined the term *aromatherapy* in the late 1930s. Modern aromatherapy traditions have evolved from *Ayurvedic* herbal uses, European and English massage, and spa traditions, and have been since adopted by holistic health and wellness centers throughout the world.

How does aromatherapy work?

When you take a whiff of aromatic vapor, the molecules enter the nasal passages where they stimulate olfactory receptor sites and trigger nerve messages to the limbic center brain. This area of the brain is thought to have evolved more than seventy million years ago and predates the neocortex, our thinking brain. Olfactory information is relayed to the amygdala in the limbic center, which is associated with emotions, memory, sleep, appetite, and sexual response. Because of these brain responses to aromas, the use of aromatherapy can enhance your joy of living by assisting with mood and emotions, memory recall, appetite, and the support of natural sleep rhythms.

How to use the oils

Essential oils can be used in a wide variety of ways, but the most common methods are by inhalation or topical use, such as lotion, body oil, or in the bath.

Inhalation

Electric micro-mist diffusers, available by mail order or at health food stores, disperse essential oils into the air in a cool mist, or they can be gently warmed in a candle heated aroma lamp that releases the aroma into the air. Adding thirty to forty drops of essential oils to a four ounce water spritz bottle is a convenient way to aromatically mist a room for immediate effect. Any essential oils you enjoy can be used for environmental fragrance; however, uplifting and energizing oils are generally used in the morning, with relaxing oils used in the late afternoon and evening. Essential oils can also be added to a special port of many room humidifiers.

There are proprietary aromatherapy inhalers similar to the familiar Vicks® Vapor Inhaler which are named by type of fragrance or identified purpose. Alternatively, you can easily put a drop or two of essential oil on your palm, rub your hands together briskly, cup them together, and breathe from your hands. You can also put several drops of essential oils on a tissue for an aromatic time out or take some sniffs directly from the bottle.

Topical Uses

Essential oils can easily be added to body lotion for use after a bath or shower, or at bedtime to prepare for sleep. Combining essential oils with touch is wonderful for calming anxiety and fears and helping to relieve exhaustion. Foot, neck, and shoulder massages are especially relaxing at bedtime and can be an enjoyable time of giving and receiving during the evening hours. For body lotion or massage oil, use about ten to fifteen drops of essential oils for each ounce of lotion or massage oil, such as grapeseed, jojoba, or apricot kernel oil.

Massage can help maintain muscle tone, improve blood circulation and lymph flow, and improve overall immune response. Seek out a massage therapist who uses aromatherapy or take your personal essential oils to be used with the massage. A refreshing aromatic body lotion can be made with six drops lavender, three drops geranium and juniper berry in an ounce of vegetable oil or lotion. (See chapter 32, *Self-massage* for more information.)

Aromatherapy baths can be an effective way to reduce the effects of emotional stress such as irritability, depression, and insomnia. Put six to ten drops of essential oils in a full tub of warm water, using a dispersing agent or surfactant such as castile soap, milk, or Epsom salts to mix the essential oils in the water. Avoid citrus rind (orange, lemon, grapefruit) and spice (cinnamon, clove) and peppermint oils in the bath as they can irritate the skin. (See chapter 34, *Water Therapy* for more information.)

Explore the variety of essential oils

There are many essential oils to choose from and aromatherapy displays offer testers for people to discover their favorite scents. Use what you and your care partner enjoy! Preferences in fragrance can vary greatly depending on past associations, gender, and personality. You might find a fragranced soap, cologne, or after shave lotion to be the perfect aromatic scent for the day. Several essential oils are known to be mood balancing or adaptogenic. These oils are versatile in their uses and can help settle restlessness or uplift malaise or depression, depending on what is needed. Examples of these oils include rose, jasmine, pink grapefruit, ylang ylang, orange, and geranium. Lavender is recommended most often for use with anxiety, agitation, and sleep.

Citrus oils are generally refreshing and uplifting for the mind and emotions, relieve stress and anxiety, and are useful for odor management and appetite support. Consider: bergamot, grapefruit, lemon, and orange.

Floral oils are often used as a personal fragrance and are useful to relieve anxiety, depression, and irritability. These oils are useful as an inhaler, in a body lotion, and for the bath. Consider: clary sage, geranium, lavender, rose, and ylang ylang.

Tree oils are revitalizing with immune boosting properties, ease respiratory congestion, and are supportive to breathing ease. They are useful for pain relief, skin infections, and odor management, and can relieve nervous exhaustion and depression. Consider: eucalyptus (*Eucalytpus citriodora* or *globulus*), pine needle, sandalwood, or Tea Tree.

Green, herbaceous, and spice oils can relieve fatigue and help circulation, digestion, pain relief, and odor management, and support the immune system. Consider: lemongrass, sweet marjoram, black pepper, peppermint, rosemary, and thyme.

Resin oils are often used for emotional and spiritual support. They can be used easily with other oils, and are known for their grounding, stress reduction, and consoling properties. Consider: frankincense and myrrh.

Root oils are earthy, emotionally calming and grounding, and are often used as fragrance and anointing oils. Consider: spikenard, patchouli, and vetiver.

Many long-term care facilities offer massage to residents. Morris regularly got an aromatherapy massage while he lived in a memory care home.

It always uplifted and relaxed him. I also put a plug-in diffuser in his room with a calming oil that contained lavender, lemon, rose geranium, marjoram, and sandalwood oils. As soon as I put a few drops on the reusable pad, inserted it into the diffuser and plugged it into the wall, Morris would deeply inhale and exclaim, "Something smells so good!" It relaxed him – and me – immediately.

Aromatherapy from early to advanced stages of Alzheimer's

An aspect of caring for an Alzheimer's patient is to reduce the level of stress as much as possible by providing an environment the care partner understands and one in which he or she feels secure. Depression frequently accompanies dementia, especially in the early stages. In more advanced stages, disorientation to time and place can occur and there are challenges completing daily living activities. Communication can be difficult and belligerent behaviors emerge. A common symptom that arises in the late phases of dementia is *sundowning*, when a person becomes confused late in the afternoon and early evening. Symptoms can include wandering and agitation, with intermittent violent behavior. Environmental supports, such as a comfortable chair, adjustable lighting, music, and an aromatherapy diffuser or mister can help.

Several Alzheimer care situations are described below where the use of aromatherapy proved to be very helpful in redirecting behavior and providing comfort.

- An agitated client in a long-term care facility wanted to "go home" and was pacing in an agitated manner. The staff put several drops of an un-named essential oil on the man's shirt collar and on the back of a nearby sofa. The gentleman soon sat on the couch, took a few deep breaths, and was able to relax and stay seated for a long time.

- A client with Alzheimer's who was in the emergency room became agitated while being wheeled to the imaging department for an MRI. The nurse put a bottle of lavender under his nose and he calmed down and allowed the technician to do the procedure.

- For a residential client with insomnia, twelve drops of lavender and patchouli were added to an ounce of water for a room spritz. The client's room and bed sheets were misted prior to his going to bed and as needed during the night. The client began having consistent restful sleep shortly afterwards.

- An aromatherapy blend of lavender and vetiver was used in a roll-on perfume applicator for an eighty-three-year-old Alzheimer's client who had insomnia, anxiety, and depression. The oil was applied to her neck and arms, and the inside of her wrists every three to four hours during the day. If the applications of aromatic oils became inconsistent her mood became increasingly anxious and agitated. As long as the essential oils were applied regularly she remained peaceful and calm.

Additional ideas using aromatherapy with care partners

- Spray citrus or floral essential oils onto a handkerchief or tissue in the morning and tuck it into a shirt pocket. Citrus and floral oils have naturally energizing and uplifting properties, and can be useful to stimulate appetite.

- Incorporate air diffusers that release essential oils such as lavender or geranium. The diffusers can be used in bathrooms to disperse relaxing scents while showering, and in sitting areas and private rooms.

- Use aromas from natural herbs and spices to trigger memories for dementia patients and their caregivers. Fill different jars with coffee beans, fresh rose petals, slices of orange rind or lemon zest, dried pineapple, cinnamon, anise, and nutmeg. Invite the care partners to smell the aromas, as well as touch the items for tactile stimulation, if appropriate. If the Alzheimer's patient is able to speak, this is a wonderful activity to initiate conversation and promote memories of the past.

- Alzheimer's and dementia patients often have poor appetites. Oils that help stimulate appetite and help with memory include many of the fruit rind and spice oils: lemon, lime, orange and grapefruit, and nutmeg, clove, cinnamon, ginger, and cardamom.

- A foot soak with relaxing essential oils can be a useful activity during times of high anxiety and restlessness. Sit with the client for added support and gentle distraction.

- Aromatic sachets can be made with porous ribbon filled with cotton, or potpourri scented with essential oils. These can be tucked into a pillow, a pocket, or left on a bedside table.

Clinical studies

Researchers at the Tottori University in Yonago, Japan studied the effects of aromatherapy in twenty-eight elderly people; seventeen had Alzheimer's disease (AD). Rosemary and lemon essential oils were used in the morning, and lavender and orange in the evening for twenty-eight days, followed by a twenty-eight day washout period (without the aromatherapy). The patients were evaluated with several cognitive assessment scales before the control period, after the control period, after aromatherapy, and after the washout period. All the patients showed significant improvement in cognitive function on the tests. The researchers concluded that aromatherapy might have some potential for improving cognitive function, especially in Alzheimer's patients.

In a study of seventy Chinese older adults with dementia, half were randomly assigned to the active group (lavender inhalation) for three weeks and then switched to control group (sunflower inhalation) for another three weeks; the other half did the opposite. Lavender was found to be effective as an adjunctive therapy in alleviating agitated behaviors in the patients with dementia. In a patient population particularly vulnerable to side effects of psychotropic medications, using lavender oil may offer an alternative option.

* * *

Laraine Pounds, *RN, MSN, BSN, CMT is the Boulder, CO Director of The Institute of Integrative Aromatherapy and Resources for Living Well, a mail order company featuring aromatherapy products.* larainekp@gmail.com, www.aroma-rn.com, www.resourcesforlivingwell.com.

* * *

References

Jimbo D, Kimura Y, Taniguchi M, Inoue M, Urakami K. "Effect of aromatherapy on patients with Alzheimer's disease." *Psychogeriatrics*. 2009 Dec;9(4):173-9.

Lin PW, Chan WC, Ng BF, Lam LC. "Efficacy of aromatherapy (Lavandula angustifolia) as an intervention for agitated behaviors in Chinese older persons with dementia: a crossover randomized trial." *International Journal of Geriatric Psychiatry*. 2007 May;22(5):405-1.

19

Art Therapy

Even if you or your care partner have never picked up a paint brush this chapter will encourage you to explore the world of art. It provides numerous ideas and art exercises and proves that simple art-making can increase relaxation and happiness.

"I found I could say things with color and shapes that I couldn't say any other way – things I had no words for."
– Georgia O'Keeffe

By **Meg Carlson**

Art therapy offers a universal channel that allows an individual to take any material, be in relationship with the material, and express feelings, emotions, and thoughts on the paper, or whatever surface that is used. Art can stimulate emotions and be the result of something that emerges unconsciously. Sometimes making art can be relieving and releasing. The artist puts feelings, emotions, and thoughts on the paper and it becomes a relief, because the feelings and thoughts are released and can reside in the texture or object. The art making becomes something that takes on its own life and is contained in its own way.

For an art therapist there are three witnesses to the art making: the therapist, the artist, and the art itself, which reflects what is present back to the artist. Art therapy offers another voice in the room, but no one needs to speak out loud. If something is hard to say, or if there is something we're not ready to face in a confrontational way, art therapy offers a safe, contained space so that an individual can express feelings, frustrations, or thoughts without having to describe them to anyone or to even understand the art that is created. There are layers of expression that we can connect with, without any of it having to make sense.

For instance, when I work with a caregiver who might have pent-up emotions, anticipatory grief from watching a loved one deteriorate, or daily stress because of things not working the way they used to, I might recommend that the person try working with water-based paints. These paints are fluid and don't impose boundaries. Using water-based paints invites emotional expression, whereas a marker drawn on a piece of paper leaves a defined mark in a contained space.

Art making helps caregivers regain a sense of balance

When a caregiver does a daily drawing, a sense of "checking-in" starts to arise. The time spent drawing or painting becomes a valuable and simple "check-in." It helps the person stay attuned to what is present, and to him or her self, in the midst of what is going on. If a caregiver is in a situation where the day is highly structured because of doctor appointments, therapy appointments, day-care, or medication schedules, and in the midst of that there's a lot of chaos, there might be some mood swings and difficulty in communicating with the care partner (memory loss person). Anything that someone chooses to do each day, such as a quick drawing or painting, will help by offering an opportunity to rebalance.

Creating a space for art

If a caregiver feels out of control, she or he can reconnect with what they can or want to do, and gain a sense of "I can do this." If a caregiver is doing these exercises on his own, I would encourage him to work in a small space by setting aside a table just for art. It could be in a family space where the care partner is present, but the idea of setting aside a space is important. If a person is overwhelmed and wants some alone time, but has to assemble the materials and find the space, sometimes that hassle can nix the project. Essentially, I'm inviting caregivers to find a space and make it sacred. Then the space is already established, the materials are in place, and everything is ready for the caregiver to make art.

As an example, when I interned at Denver Hospice on a Sunday afternoon or morning, I'd tape a 6x6 piece of paper on a table. I had a drawer full of art materials and a cup of water. Sometimes twice a day, I'd go to that piece of paper and add to it what I needed to. The space was already prepared, so I didn't have to look for the materials. They were there to help me refresh myself.

Helping care partners reconnect

I worked with a married couple in which the man had severe dementia. He couldn't talk, other than make sounds and nonsensical words. He often would just stare at things. First, just he and I did art, so his wife could get things done around the house. Their interactions were difficult, so I invited her to come make art with us.

The couple had traveled extensively during their marriage, so we did collages using pictures of where they'd been. The husband would look at them and connect with the pictures, and then they'd connect with each other. It was very bittersweet because it brought up a lot of good memories. It also became clear that the wife had so much anticipatory grief (a feeling of loss before a death or dreaded event occurs).

The husband

The husband had been a preacher, and he loved to listen to recordings of music from the church where he had worked. His cognitive ability improved while he listened to that music, so we started using watercolors on large pieces of paper while he listened. I put down tape on the paper in different shapes and directions; a process used by painters called "cutting." Cutting is easy for someone who has difficulty making shapes because when the tape is removed, there are nicely cut, really clean shapes left on the surface.

Before the tape was removed, sometimes the preacher would dip the brush in the paint and we'd paint the shapes. After the tape was removed, he was left with a windowpane that reminded him of stained glass windows. I don't know if he felt a sense of accomplishment, but he'd spend time looking at and pointing to the miniature stained glass windows. He'd share it with his wife and me. It was a beautiful learning process.

The wife

The husband had a habit of clearing items off every table in the house, but the wife found a solution to creating a private space for making art. She taped a piece of paper onto a window and kept art materials and markers on top of the refrigerator. That way she knew she always had the space and materials available and she didn't have to worry about her husband's other habit of hiding her things.

The wife would add to the piece of paper throughout the day; whatever was pertinent to how or what she was feeling. She found that having a safe, sacred space, even though it was just on a windowpane and on top of the refrigerator, offered her a great relief from stress.

Helping caregivers deal with grief

When the wife did water colors or the collage with her husband, she'd share stories, which helped her husband interact with us. The activity reduced her stress and increased her ability to be present with her husband, and it also addressed her anticipatory grief and triggered her sense of loss. She was able to reflect on joyful things they had shared and on what had been lost. For her, making art was about accessing the grief and expressing it.

Art therapy helps caregivers reflect on their grief and some of the things that have been lost. Even though the person they are caring for is still there, the creation of a mandala, drawing, or a shape allows each caregiver to be more present with their care partner. They can honor the grief that arises in small increments, on a day-to-day basis. This supports the caregivers and helps to keep emotions from compounding until they feel impossible to express.

What I've learned by working with families in which someone has dementia is that the loss is there every day. It accumulates and becomes overwhelming. Caregivers are often surprised to have strong feelings arise while making a meal or doing something very ordinary. Feelings and recognition of loss might happen on a day-to-day basis, offering the opportunity to reflect on and name what's going on, including both the joys and losses. Caring for someone who has memory loss is unique, because the caregiving extends over many years and the loss happens in small increments. A caregiver might realize one afternoon that *"today I need to change all the light bulbs."* It sounds simple, but recognizing that her husband is not there to help anymore, that her partner is here but not really here, is one of the small, subtle things that contribute to anticipatory grief.

Building a life with someone you love is made up of a lot of subtle things that fit together. We're individuals, but we connect in so many ways. Having a partner that loses his or her cognitive functioning is an undoing of all those subtle agreements that you've made together. It shows how small things make up what's so amazing about being in a relationship.

Art making with people with memory loss

The goal of making art with someone who is memory impaired is to engage with that person and provide an experience of accomplishment and enjoyment. The parameters about putting too many colors on the page or coloring inside the lines dissolve. When I work with folks in assisted living, we do group projects and the people get excited and have a sense of accomplishment. Since the empty page is unnerving for some people, I provide some structure by handing out beautiful black and white images from high-end coloring books. Regardless of what the person chooses to do, we frame it and put their name on it.

One time, I asked people to color an image of a dog. The picture evolved depending on the person's cognitive ability, but none of that mattered. Most of them were able to fool around with the image and relate to it. People started to share about the dog image and that alone became a fun experience. One person said, "I used to have a dog," which led to a lively group discussion about family pets.

I worked with one woman who used to be a painter. She was very physically fit, and could go on epic walks, but she'd get confused. She'd always ask for a piece of clean paper and then she'd access her inner artist and paint beautiful flowers and large, gorgeous roses. She remembered that she used to be an artist and was excited about it.

Some people get nervous about creating art, especially the ones who have never worked with art materials. The key is to find a relaxed place and just begin by having the person find his or her favorite colors. Then stories, images, and colors emerge.

After the assisted living folks did their art projects, we'd display them in an art exhibit and share them with family members. That was also a neat process. A few people felt it was childish, but the art was unique to each person and everyone felt a sense of pride. The biggest thing to remember is that, even though the goals have changed, care partners can feel a sense of accomplishment and enjoyment. The goal is to have a good time.

Art exercises for caregivers

1. Making an Inside/Outside Box

Materials:

- Boxes-shoe box, tea box, metal tin, etc.
- Mixed media-crayons, paint, markers, glue, feathers, felt, rocks, etc.

Decorating a box allows the artist to reflect his or her persona or face that is shown to the outside world on the outside of the box. Decorating the inside of the box is an opportunity to express the internal feelings and conflicts that are private or feel too big to find words to express. Use whatever materials that are available to decorate the outside of the box and then the inside of the box to express these feelings.

Outside Box: How do you experience being around others with your loved one? What do you share with the outside world about your process and how do you share?

Inside Box: What is really going on inside of you each day? What isn't shared with others that has an impact on you?

What has this process, or your imagery, expressed to you? What kinds of responses are you having?

2. *Daily or Weekly Mandalas*

A mandala is a circular image. It begins with a circle drawn on a page. It can be any size and any medium can be used.

Materials/Time:

- Paper: Bristol, Watercolor, or mixed media (6x6 is a great size)
- Pencils, markers, watercolor, colored pencil, pastels, or crayons are all great.

It is small enough to be done in a brief sitting and large enough to have room for several images or areas of focus.

A version of mandalas exists in many spiritual traditions (rose windows in Cathedrals, Navajo and Tibetan sand paintings, Buddhist imagery). Mandalas can be used to support focusing attention, as a self-check-in tool, to express emotions in a contained space (circle), for establishing a sacred space, and to aid in mindfulness and meditation. Carl Jung, through his own art process, came to realize that mandala paintings enabled him to identify dysfunctional emotional patterns and work towards integration and wholeness.

3. *Color-Texture-Pattern Feelings Portrait*

This process is about awareness of how much is going on in each of us at any given moment. It is an opportunity to just *GET IT OUT* through color, movement, and expression. The imagery is usually abstract. It is the process of expressing that is beneficial here, not the finished product. Feelings are difficult to identify, and when they are expressed visually they can be difficult to look at. But that is okay. If you use this process, when you are finished, take a moment to witness it like a loving friend. Then just set it aside. If your image invites a redo or edit, you can come back to it and work with it, even tear it up and re-create it. If not, let it go. The materials will support you to express emotions and that is their purpose sometimes — to help you create something that is not necessarily pretty, but honest. That is their gift to you.

Materials/Time:

- Small to medium paper. Mixed media paper is sturdy. Taped to a surface is best. When you prep, ask yourself, *"What size is my expression today?"* That will tell you what paper size to use.
- Pencils, markers, watercolor, colored pencil, pastels, or crayons are all great.

This can be done between five and twenty-five minutes. It is simply the process of choosing colors and making textures and patterns that express the layers of your feelings. Let the speed and movement be an extension of your expression. It will be unique every time.

4. Two-Inch Window Drawing

The goal is to work with detail and discernment to create a bird's eye view. Another way to use this tool is one of magnification; to zoom in to one aspect of something larger. An example could be to feel a single sensation, filling a small (contained) space with just what is magnified. Used as a daily or coping practice, it may serve to redirect concentration or focus energy and attention, or provide containment while titrating an intense sensation. They take between one and ten minutes to complete. Think Macro and Micro — what would be most helpful to step back or lean in?

Materials/Time:

- Paper: Bristol, watercolor, or mixed media (2x2 or 4x4)
- Card stock scraps come in several colors, and can usually be found at craft stores.

This drawing is small enough to be done in a brief sitting and can even be a single set of colors.

5. Process: Journey Drawing

Materials:

- Paper: Bristol, watercolor, or mixed media (6x6 or larger)
- Collage materials, or a material you enjoy (fabric, craft papers, natural materials, etc.)

- Chalk/oil pastels, pencil, watercolor

Where are you in this journey? Emotionally — physically — personally — socially? Is there stuckness? Is there movement? What colors, shapes, textures represent where you are right now? What colors feel supportive of your journey or give you strength? What emotions are present for you about your current life, about being a caregiver? Can you think of any supportive guides/helpers that you have met along the way? How has your identity or personality been challenged or changed in this process? Who in your life is accepting these changes? Who is having difficulty accepting the changes?

What has this process, or your imagery, expressed to you? If you had a chance to respond to it, what kinds of responses are you having? Are you in a different place in your journey than you assumed/thought/hoped? What are the qualities of where you feel you are in your journey as a caregiver? As you have moved through different stages, what has each stage offered you?

Lastly, choose a color that feels strengthening, a color that will help you move into the next stage of your journey. Now create a final piece of your drawing that will offer you strength and power when you look at it. Be one of the helpers for yourself in this moment of your journey.

6. Process: Breath Drawing

Materials:

- Oil pastels or chalk pastels
- Large paper
- Your breath
  Draw your breath with one color in each hand. Notice the qualities of your inhale (short, stunted, deep, long, interrupted, fast, shallow) and allow your hands and the colors to express it. Do the same with the exhale. What are the qualities present in your out breath? Move each hand/ arm in a circular motion with the expression and notice how the lines change over time. Notice similarities and any shifts. Follow your own breath with soft awareness.

What has this process, or your imagery, expressed to you? What kinds of responses are you having?

* * *

Meg Carlson, MA, LPAT has worked in the field of Art Therapy since 2010, both in agencies and in private practice. She graduated from Naropa University with a master's degree in Transpersonal Counseling and Art Therapy. Meg is dedicated to sharing and teaching about the therapeutic qualities of art and bridging the knowledge of art practices and therapeutic techniques. She can be reached at: art.m.carlson@gmail.com.

Memories in the Making® Art Making Program

Memories in the Making® originated at the Alzheimer's Association Orange County (CA) Chapter in 1988. The program was developed by Selly Jenny, whose mother had Alzheimer's disease. Selly wanted to create a meaningful activity that would have a positive impact on the physical, mental, and emotional health of people with dementia, and would encourage them to freely express themselves. Today, the program is in memory care facilities and adult day care programs throughout the United States. It is estimated there are more than four thousand artists participating in a *Memories in the Making®* Art Program each week.

Interview with Denver Artist Lisa Hut

I volunteer for the Alzheimer's Association and facilitate a *Memories in the Making®* (MIM) watercolor painting class with dementia patients once a week. The program, which is art making and not art therapy, encourages communication through painting, increasing self-esteem, and providing sensory stimulation. Individuals with dementia are often able to paint memories or emotions that they can no longer communicate. The program has a high level of integrity (using archival watercolor paints & paper), and truly gives patients that are losing all sense of communication a way to communicate.

I've facilitated this class at nursing homes and an Assisted Living Care Community. It is supposed to be one hour long, but since

I currently have high functioning people, sometimes we go for three hours. I love, love, love this program! I am so lucky that I can use my passion for art in such a wonderful volunteer capacity. Memories often come up from doing something like painting. I try to give small prompts and ask the participants if their painting reminds them of anything. But one hundred percent of the artwork is the artist's work. If they can't quite dip the brush into the water, we'll help them. But we never guide their hand or do a pre-sketch. Family members are always welcome to sit and do their own painting. We encourage the people in the class to title their paintings without our help, and I try not to put words in their mouth when they are trying to come up with a title.

One day I was working with a man named Ray who was non-verbal and low functioning. I sat down with him, showed him a calendar picture of a sunset, and asked him to paint bright colors from left to right across the page. When I told Ray, "This is a beautiful sunset you've painted," he spewed out a story about being in the navy and stationed on the USS Saratoga in San Diego during WWII. He said that a plane had landed on the ship and that his acquaintance was killed the next day. (Ray had lost the word for friend.)

With Alzheimer's, so much of the person is lost and gone, and sometimes the stories they tell aren't necessarily true and get jumbled up with their memories. But when families come in, frequently the title of the painting becomes a jumping-off point for reminiscing. And sometimes a family member will confirm that the story that emerged from their loved one's painting is indeed true.

Every time we paint, there are bittersweet moments; a little bit of crying and a little bit of laughing. The painters have a great sense of humor. Once a man painted a picture of a horse and started talking about a horse that would push a baby around in a buggy. The family confirmed that he had lived on a farm where this was a frequent event, and they brought in an old photo of the horse and the baby inside the buggy to prove it.

After we paint all year, we collect the artwork and have an annual art auction. Professional painters are invited to view the paintings and, if they like one, they'll do a pairing where they generously donate one of their paintings to hang next to a *Memories in the Making®* painting. We have approximately one hundred pieces

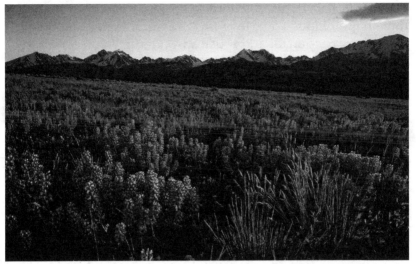

Lupine, Gore Range, Colorado.
Photo by John Fielder. See the full color image at <u>barbracohn.com</u>.

of art painted by people with Alzheimer's disease or some other form of dementia, and between thirty and thirty-five professional artists who participate. The paintings that are paired with pieces from professionals have sold from $2,000 up to $10,000. Smaller individual paintings and painted palettes sell from fifty dollars. All the money raised at the art auction is donated to the Alzheimer's Association. The Colorado Chapter raised $400,000 in 2013 from art auctions.

A woman named Bettie did a painting that she titled "*God's Beauty.*" It was very colorful and bright with bursts of purple. John Fielder, the well-known nature photographer, donated a similar mountain scene with grasses in the foreground titled "*Gore Range, Lupine, Summit County, Colorado.*" He framed his photograph and Bettie's painting in the same frame, which is what he always does for the art shows. The family was absolutely thrilled since they were long time admirers of John Fielder's work.

Bettie's son Barry Van Zetten added, "My mother has always been passionate about painting and dreamed about becoming an artist. She did some metal sculptures in her spare time, and sold a few paintings at consignment shops, so it's cool to see her dream come full circle. But it's a little tragic that she doesn't realize that this painting was paired with John Fielder's photograph and sold at the auction."

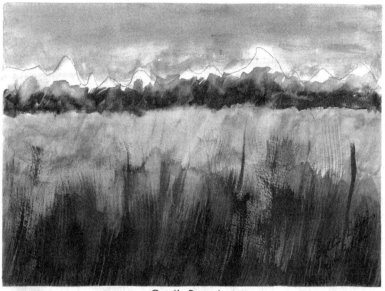

God's Beauty.
by Bettie Van Zetten. See the full color image at barbracohn.com

Every January we have a meeting at the Alzheimer's Association Colorado Chapter's office in Denver to view the art that's been chosen for the show. The attending volunteers and care community employees that facilitate the class share many heartfelt stories. One person told us that after an elderly patient died, the family came to pick up the belongings and were unaware that their loved one had participated in MIM. The art was all tied up with a ribbon and they were stunned to have this legacy of art. They turned the art over and saw all the titles and stories written on the back and were very deeply moved. All the volunteers and employees were in tears.

It's important to note that the *Memories in the Making*® program focuses on painting for the process and the experience, not the end results ... because the end results — whether simple or abstract — are wonderful paintings. My feeling is that when you have dementia you are constantly messing up and doing things the wrong way. Ordinarily, folks with dementia are afraid of making a social mistake. But when we paint together, these same people are completely relaxed and their stress goes away because we emphasize that there is nothing they can do wrong when they are painting.

If they are reluctant to put brush to paper, I say, "Oh, come in and sit down. I'm going to help you." They completely enjoy the process and it's a great stress reliever. Since we use one hundred and forty pound archival paper that will last forever, along with high quality watercolors, I can talk to them at a higher level about their work, since I'm an artist. The intention is that they are working as real artists. We welcome anyone to come in and observe or help. You can see how much I love this program!

* * *

Lisa Hut has been an artist for as long as she can remember. She studied at the Art Institute of Dallas and worked as a graphic designer for twelve years. She taught art while her children were young and always had an art project on hand. When her aunt was diagnosed with Alzheimer's disease in 2008, Lisa started volunteering with the Memories in the Marking Art Program. "Every single week there have been heartfelt, bittersweet moments, lots of laughter, and sometimes tears. But I can't wait to go back next week."

* * *

References

Jung, C. G, *Memories, Dreams, Reflections* (New York: Random House, 1989).

20

Ayurveda

A̶yurveda, the oldest health care system in the world, emerged from India thousands of years ago. In this chapter, renowned Ayurvedic physician, Dr. John Douillard describes the basic tenets and explains how to determine your body type. Dietary and lifestyle recommendations are made accordingly to improve your digestion, quality of sleep, and to support a balanced physiology. Individuals may find that adopting an Ayurvedic lifestyle helps their ability to stay strong and keep their care partners more relaxed and content.

"Ayurveda is useful for everyone because the main objective of Ayurveda is to preserve and maintain health. Those who are healthy will benefit from Ayurveda by becoming stronger and having more energy; while those who are sick will be able to bring back their health in a natural way." – Dr. Vasant Lad

Ayurveda: The Ancient Vedic Science That Helps Restore Balance and Prevent Illness

By Dr. **John Douillard**

Ayurveda is a Sanskrit word derived from two roots: *ayur*, which means life, and *veda*, which means knowledge. It has its root in ancient Vedic science and encompasses our entire world — nature, the body, mind, and spirit. Ayurveda focuses on prevention of illness and the body's natural power to heal itself.

History and basic principles

Ayurvedic medical texts date back to 2500 B.C. According to the ancient texts, there are five elements that compose everything in the universe, including the human body: earth, water, fire, air, and sky/ether. Within the human body there are seven layers, called *dhatus,* which get treated: plasma, blood, flesh, fat, bone, marrow, semen or female reproductive tissue.

Body type

In Ayurveda there are three main body types also known as *doshas*: Vata, Pitta, and Kapha. These body types are reflections of the qualities of nature. They give insight, not just into the tendencies of our bodies, but of our mental, emotional, and behavioral characteristics as well. According to Ayurvedic medicine, prevention of disease is dictated by the unique requirements of your body type. Because we are unique, what we eat, how we exercise, when we sleep, and even where we prefer to live, will be different from one person to the next. The best and most healthful practices for each individual can be better understood by knowing your body type.

To find out what body type you are, visit Dr. John Douillard's website and take the Body Type Quiz: lifespa.com/health-quizzes/body-type-quiz

1. Vata Constitution

Vata is the most important of the three doshas. If left unbalanced it causes Pitta and Kapha to become imbalanced.

Vata is the main driver or mover of the body, providing the following functions:

- All eliminations: fetus, semen, feces, urine, and sweat
- Assists with metabolisms in the body (Agni), transformation of tissues
- Controls movement in the body (mental and physical), such as respiration, heartbeat, motivation, contraction of muscles, and natural urges
- Relays all sensory input to the brain and motor functions
- Governs the nervous system

Vata: Dry, Cold
Elements: Air and Ether

Vata Body Type:

1. Small frame, light and thin / hard to gain weight
2. Course, dry, kinky or curly hair
3. Dry, rough, darker skin
4. Small eyes, whites of eyes are blue or brown
5. Very large or small teeth, crooked or shaded
6. Performs activity quickly, can't stay idle, has a quick walking pace
7. Low strength and endurance
8. Quick minded, restless, learns fast and forgets fast, high pitch / fast voice
9. Moods change quickly, tendency to worry, easily excitable, easily stressed
10. Irregular hunger and digestion, tendency towards constipation
11. Aversion to cold weather
12. Prefers warm food and drink; eats quickly
13. Spends money quickly; doesn't save
14. Variable, irregular sex drive
15. Light, interrupted sleep; dreams are fearful, flying, jumping, and running

Symptoms of Imbalance

- Dry or rough skin
- Insomnia
- Constipation
- Fatigue
- Headaches

- Intolerance of cold
- Underweight or losing weight
- Anxiety, worry, and restlessness
- Attention Deficit with Hyperactivity Disorder

It's especially easy for Vata to get out of balance during winter.

To balance Vata

- Favor foods that are warm, heavy, oily, sweet, sour, and salty
- Eat three warm, nourishing meals each day
- Pay attention to fluids, avoid cold or iced drinks, sip warm water at regular intervals; avoid alcoholic beverages, coffee, and black tea
- In winter include savory squash soup, stews, steamed veggies, and warm herbal teas

2. Pitta Constitution

Wherever there is transformation, there is Pitta.

Pitta provides the following functions:

- Metabolism — from digestion of food to transformation of all other material
- Thermogenesis — maintains the proper body temperature
- Vision
- Comprehension of information into knowledge / reasoning and judgment
- Complexion — gives color and softness to skin

Pitta: Hot, Moist (Oily), Light
Elements: Fire and Water

Pitta Body Type

- Medium frame, medium weight
- Thin, lustrous hair with fine curls
- Soft, medium oily, pink to red skin
- Penetrating eyes, whites of eyes are yellow or red
- Small to medium yellowish teeth
- Average walking pace, competitive
- Good strength and endurance
- Sharp intellect, aggressive, good general memory, medium pitch / clear voice
- Slow changing moods, angers easily, quick temper, likes things to be orderly
- Sharp hunger, can't miss a meal, good digestion, normal elimination
- Aversion to dry and hot weather
- Prefers cold food and drinks, and eats at an easy pace
- Saves money, but is a big spender
- Moderate sex drive
- Sound, medium length sleep, dreams are fiery, violent, and angry

Symptoms of Imbalance

- Rashes
- Inflammatory skin conditions (including acne)
- Stomach aches
- Diarrhea
- Controlling and manipulative behavior
- Visual problems or burning in the eyes
- Excessive body heat
- Hostility, irritability
- Excessive competitive drive

It's especially easy for Pitta to get out of balance during summer.

To balance Pitta

- Favor foods that are bitter*, sweet, and astringent*
- Drink a lot of fluids and use cool compresses in hot weather
- Eat largest meal at midday
- Decrease stimulants—avoid alcohol, coffee, and tea
- Reduce foods that are spicy, hot, salty, and sour
- To stay cool in summer, drink coconut water and smoothies, and eat more salads and fresh fruit
- Use sesame, coconut, and sunflower oils

3. Kapha Constitution

Kapha is the heaviest of the three doshas. It provides the structures and the lubrication that the body needs.

Kapha provides the following functions:

- Strength and energy
- Moistness and lubrication
- Stability to add the necessary grounding aspect to both mind and body
- Mass and structure to provide fullness to bodily tissues
- Fertility and virility

Kapha: Cold, Moist (Oily), Heavy
Elements: Water and Earth

Kapha Body Type

- Large frame, heavy, easy to gain weight
- Thick, straight / wavy, oily hair
- Oily, moist, pale, white skin
- Large eyes, whites of eyes are glossy and white
- Medium to large, white and strong teeth
- Slow and steady walking pace

- Excellent strength and endurance
- Calm, steady disposition, long-term memory, low pitch / resonating voice
- Steady, non-changing moods, slow to get irritated, very understanding, easy-going
- Can miss a meal easily, digestion can be a little slow; elimination is heavy, slow, thick and regular
- Aversion to damp and cold weather
- Prefers dry food and eats slowly
- Saves money regularly and accumulates wealth
- Strong sex drive
- Sound, heavy, and long sleep; dreams of water, clouds, and romance

Symptoms of Imbalance

- Oily skin
- Slow digestion
- Sinus congestion
- Nasal allergies
- Asthma
- Obesity
- Skin growths
- Possessiveness, neediness
- Depression
- Difficulty paying attention
- Apathy

It is especially easy for Kapha to get out of balance during spring.

To balance Kapha

- Eat more foods that are pungent (spicy), bitter*, astringent** / light, dry, warm: such as flavorful steamed veggies, brothy soups, brown rice

- Eat fewer foods that are sweet, sour, salty / heavy, cold, oily: such as fried foods, ice cream, heavy dairy
- Use sesame and olive oils

  *Bitter foods and spices include: turmeric, fenugreek seeds, leafy greens, barley, basil, lettuce, jicama

  **Astringent foods include: apple, pear, quinoa, legumes, tofu, beans, lentils

Ayurvedic recommendations for healthy living

Live according to the natural cycles. Ayurveda recommends following these guidelines — as discussed in Dr. Douillard's book *The 3-Season Diet*, (Three Rivers Press 2000) — in order to align yourself with the natural cycles:

- Arise at, or before, sunrise. Sleeping in increases more tiredness and stiffness.
- Engage in some practice of exercise in the morning. This is a great time for yoga, breathing, and meditation as a regular part of the daily routine. It's also the best time of day for a cardiovascular workout.
- Be careful not to overeat at breakfast.
- Make lunch the biggest meal of the day, and create a relaxed environment.
- Strive to include seasonal foods.
- Rest for 10-15 minutes after lunch; even a short nap, lying on your left side after this meal is okay.
- Evaluate how you feel in the afternoon.
- If you have cravings, try to make lunch a more satisfying and balanced meal.
- If you tend to crash in the afternoon, adhere to the above guidelines. Convenience foods that are eaten quickly will be difficult to digest, and will not deliver the fuel your brain demands at this time.
- Meditate between 5 p.m.-6 p.m. If this is not realistic for your schedule, carve out at least sixty seconds and try a One Minute Meditation. Dr. Douillard teaches this

technique at: lifespa.com/one-minute-meditation/#. Ukmt6byE7cE

- Avoid eating heavy meals late in the day. Eat light and early.

- Exercise is okay between 6 p.m.-7 p.m., but not later because it could over-stimulate you and disturb your sleep.

- Start settling down for the evening as early as possible. The habit of staying up late is difficult to change, but getting to bed early is essential for longevity and increased cognitive function as you age.

- If you have difficulty settling down, try an Ojas nightly tonic before bed. For more information visit: store.lifespa. com

- Eat early so you are finished digesting by the time you go to sleep.

- Exercise early so the body's cortisol and adrenaline levels are not stimulated at night, which can affect sleep and nighttime liver detoxification.

- Consider meditating or reading a relaxing book before bed. Good old-fashioned bedtime stories work well!

- Get to sleep before 10 p.m..

- Over time, after getting to bed early and eating supper early, you will naturally begin to wake up earlier. This will happen without an alarm and, although you might still have to end the habit of sleeping in, the body will no longer need that extra rest.

* * *

John Douillard DC is the author of six books, including The 3-Season Diet: Eat the Way Nature Intended *(Three Rivers Press, 2000) and has published more than four hundred health videos and articles, and numerous health DVDs and CDs. He has formulated his own line of organic health care products. Dr. Douillard co-directed Deepak Chopra's Ayurvedic Center for eight years before founding and directing the LifeSpa Ayurvedic Retreat Center in Boulder, CO where he lives with his wife and six children. 1-866-227-9843;* lifespa.com.

* * *

Ayurvedic herb for brain and nerve support

Bacopa monnieria, also known as Brahmi, is the most potent and effective nerve and brain tonic in Ayurvedic medicine. It has been used for centuries to help people of all ages learn and remember new information. It has also been traditionally used to treat mental illness, anxiety, depression, memory loss, epilepsy, and psychosis. In ancient Vedic texts, Bacopa is classified as a *rasayana* (herbal remedy) to slow down brain aging and help regenerate neural tissues. Today, Ayurvedic doctors use it to support cognitive and attention issues.

Bacopa supports memory

A 2002 study published in the journal *Neuropsychopharmacology* found that using Bacopa monnieri for three months might improve memory. When seventy-six participants were tested on retention of new information, the placebo group forgot the information more quickly than the group taking Bacopa.

Bacopa supports cognitive performance and reduces anxiety and depression

Bacopa helps reduce anxiety and depression in the elderly. In a double-blind placebo controlled study at Helfgott Research Institute, National College of Natural Medicine in Portland, Oregon, forty-eight participants, sixty-five or older, were given a daily dose of three hundred mg. of Bacopa or a placebo for twelve weeks.

The participants did not have clinical signs of dementia, but those who took Bacopa showed improved word recall memory scores in comparison to the placebo group. The Bacopa group also showed less anxiety and depression after taking the supplement when compared to the placebo group.

Bacopa decreases stress

In addition to the improved cognitive function reported by the Portland study, which appeared in the *Journal of Alternative and Complementary Medicine*, the participants taking Bacopa showed fewer mood issues. It's also interesting that heart rate decreased in the Bacopa group over time, but increased in the placebo group.

How does Bacopa work?

A number of compounds have been identified in Bacopa, including bacosides A and B—two chemicals that improve the transmission of impulses between nerve cells in the brain. These bacosides support cognitive function, making it easier to learn and remember new information. Bacopa also supports the neurotransmitter acetylcholine (important for learning and memory), and serotonin and GABA (gamma amiobutyric acid), neurotransmitters that promote relaxation.

How safe is Bacopa?

Bacopa is safe and effective for people of all ages, without any known side effects. It does not contain addictive ingredients and can be used indefinitely.

Recipe for kitcheree

Kitcheree is wonderfully comforting for colds, flu, stomach upset, and recovery from surgery. Enjoy year-round for an easy-to-digest, nutritious, one-pot meal.

Kitcheree for two (Thanks to David Rose)

- 4 Tbsp organic Basmati rice
- 4 Tbsp mung dahl (can use red or yellow lentils)
- 4 ½ cups water (more or less, depending on whether you like it soupy or thick)
- 2 tsp grated fresh ginger
- 2 Tbsp fresh lemon juice
- 1 cup assorted veggies, cut into bite-sized pieces: yam, carrot, potato, cauliflower, broccoli—your choice
- salt and pepper to taste
- optional: fresh chopped cilantro or parsley
- 1 tsp ground coriander seed
- 1 ½ tsp ghee

- ¼ tsp brown mustard seeds

Combine the rice, dahl, ginger, veggies, and water in a pot. Add coriander. Bring to a boil over medium heat; then lower the heat and simmer, partially covered, for about 45-50 minutes, occasionally stirring. Add water if it gets too thick. Remove from the stove. Heat the ghee in a small saucepan over medium high heat. Add the mustard seeds and cover. When the seeds have all popped, remove from the stove and add to the kitcheree. Add the lemon juice, salt and pepper, and cilantro or parsley.

Enjoy a feast in a pot!

* * *

References

Bhattacharya, S., A Kumar, A. Ghosal. 2000. "Effect of Bacopa monniera on animal models of Alzheimer's disease and perturbed central cholinergic markers of cognition in rats." In: Sanka, Siva. *Molecular Aspects of Asian Medicine.* (New York: PJD Publications, 2000).

Bone, Kerry, Carlo Calabrese, William L. Gregory, Dale Kraemer, Michael Leo, and Barry Oken. 2008. "Effect of Bacopa monniera on animal models of Alzheimer's disease and perturbed central cholinergic markers of cognition in rats." *Journal of Alternative and Complementary Medicine.* 14(6): 707-713.

Booth, Dianne, Sonia Bulzomi, Caroline Micallef, Andrew Phipps, Steven Roodenrys, and Jaclyn Smoker. 2002. "Chronic effects of Brahmi (Bacopa monnieri) on human memory." *Neuropsychopharmacology.* 27: 279-81.

Datta, C. and PK Dey. 1966. "Effect of psychotropic phytochemicals on cerebral amino acid level in mice." *Indiana Journal of Experimental Biology.* 4(4): 216-9. Dhawan, Bhola Nath, and Singh HK. 1997. "Neuropsychopharmacological effects of the Ayurvedic nootropic Bacopa monniera Linn." *Indian Journal of Pharmacology.* 29(5): 359-36.

Dhawan, Bhola Nath, Hemant K. Singh, R.C. Srimal, and R.P. Rastogi. 2006. "Effect of bacosides A and B on avoidance responses in rats." *Phytotherapy Research.* 2(2): 70-75.

Downey, Luke Andrew, CW Hutchison, Clarke J., Jenny Lloyd, Con KK Stough. 2001. "The chronic effects of an extract of Bacopa monniera (Brahmi) on cognitive function in healthy human subjects." *Psychopharmacology.* 156(4): 481-4.

Ganguly, DK and CL Malhotra. 1967. "Some neuropharmacological and behavioral effects of an activefraction from Herpestis monniera Linn (Brahmi)." *Indian journal of physiology and pharmacology.* 11(1): 33-43.

Chapter 21

Breath Work

*B*reathe. *It's easy to forget to when you're anxious about your care partner's health, or when you haven't had enough sleep, or when you're feeling any range of emotions like guilt or anger. Relearn how to breathe with invaluable exercises that you can do by yourself and with your care partner. Your body and mind will thank you.*

"Breath is the king of mind." – B.K.S. Iyengar, *Light on Yoga*

By Reverend **Shanthi Behl**

The process by which we deliberately alter our breathing is sometimes called breath work. In yoga, it is called *pranayama*, or guidance of the *prana*. *Prana* is the energy that animates all life and we can consciously guide that energy using two subtle mechanisms.

Breath work is the first and easiest to start with. We can deliberately extend, shorten, retain, and otherwise direct the air we breathe in a variety of ways in order to guide the *prana*. Second, is the mechanism of directed attention, also known as our intention. Where our thoughts go, our *prana* goes. An integrated *pranayama* practice utilizes both the breath and our focused attention.

When we say we are tired and have no energy, what we are really saying is that our energy is blocked. We need to breathe to live, and how we breathe can profoundly affect our degree of physical well-being; it can regulate our emotions, and it can deplete, sustain, or increase our experience of aliveness. *Prana* is constantly fluctuating and moving throughout the universe. According to yoga philosophy, it flows throughout the living body in exquisitely determined whirlpools and currents. The wonderment of the yogic system is *asana* and *pranayama* practice which allows our innate energy currents to flow as nature intended.

Here is a lovely *pranayama* practice to use with an agitated individual who is "sundowning." You may be familiar with this phenomenon. Mayo Clinic clinical neuropsychologist, Glenn Smith, PhD, describes sundowning as a state of confusion at the end of the day and into the night. Sundowning isn't a disease, but a symptom that often occurs in people with dementia, such as Alzheimer's disease. Smith lists several factors that may aggravate late-day confusion including fatigue, low lighting, increased shadows, and the disease's disruption of the body's internal clock. You might find that focusing your loved one's attention on this practice calms them—and you.

Read these instructions slowly out loud as you demonstrate the movement.

- *Let us do the Butterfly Breath together.*
- *Face palms toward the heart center at center of the chest. Interlace the fingers with thumb pointing up to the ceiling. Place hands on the chest and keep your awareness at this heart center as you breathe deeply and slowly in and out the nose.*
- *Can you feel your heart beating? Can you feel how much you are loved?*
- *Notice the rise and fall of your breath. Feel the warmth of your hands on your chest.*

Add this option for yourself:

- *Notice any feelings or thoughts as you breathe naturally.*
- *As you breathe in, see your feelings and thoughts like bubbles of air rising from the bottom of a lake.*
- *Breathe out, and imagine the bubbles silently bursting as they reach the water's surface.*

Now, let us take a moment, right now, to feel our own energy. The following instructions are for sitting, but you can practice this exercise while standing in mountain pose.

- *Sit up tall, lengthen the spine, and place the feet flat on the floor. Press the feet into the ground, even as you press the top of the head toward the ceiling.*

- Relax the hands lightly on the lap and release the shoulders down away from the ears.

- Soften the belly muscles. As you breathe in through the nose, lengthen through the crown of the head.

- As you breathe out through the nose, release the shoulders and press your feet into the floor.

- Continue this practice and turn your awareness to sensations along the spinal column. Feel the upward flow as you breathe in and the downward flow as you breathe out. It is perfectly fine if you feel the opposite movement. The important aspect is to tune into a sense of any movement along the spine. You may not initially feel the movement of your energy. However, by first imagining it, you will later actually feel the upward and downward flows of energy along sushumna, the central core of energy.

* * *

Reverend **Sharon Shanthi Behl**, MA, LPC, E-RYT-500©, is ordained and credentialed as a teacher through Integral Yoga, founded by Sri Swami Satchidananda. Shanthi is a founding Board member of Yoga Alliance, Board Emeritus of Yoga Teachers of Colorado and former Advisory Board member of Rocky Mountain Institute of Yoga and Ayurveda. Shanthi provides yoga instruction to hospice patients and their caregivers by integrating contemporary Western psychology with yoga's profound wisdom. She can be reached at: peacepug2@hotmail.com.

Chapter 22

Dance

An "Einstein Aging Study" found that dance is the best physical activity to help prevent dementia. Find out why the amazing power of dance is a healing aid and how it can enhance your mood and create bliss. You'll even find a list of music and some simple instructions to help you move your body and share a sweet moment with your care partner.

Dance, when you're broken open.
Dance, if you've torn the bandage off.
Dance in the middle of the fighting.
Dance in your blood.
Dance, when you're perfectly free.
Struck, the dancers hear a tambourine inside them,
as a wave turns to foam on its very top, begin.
Maybe you don't hear that tambourine,
or the tree leaves clapping time.
Close the ears on your head
that listen mostly to lies and cynical jokes.
There are other things to hear and see:
dance-music and a brilliant city inside the Soul.
– Rumi

Dancing with Life

By **Melissa Michaels**

Across culture and time, dance has been a universal way for individuals and communities to heal, to celebrate, and to awaken. Whether it is waltzing in a ballroom with one's beloved, boogying to the radio in the living room, whirring around in one's wheel chair, or creatively expressing oneself in wild abandon, dance is something everyone can do. The truth is that everyone is a dancer. With each tap of a foot, wiggle of a finger, and sway of a hip, a dance begins. As one body part moves, other parts of our being also inevitably mobilize. Dance is a doorway into connection with one's senses, sensations, feelings, and even one's soul. Thus, the beauty of movement for Alzheimer's patients is that it actively helps these individuals literally get out of their minds and into the vast landscape of their whole beings.

Let's start with the body. Dancing is a readily available way to exercise. By moving the body, our organs, muscles, bones, and yes, our brains are nourished. Trauma patterns of flight, fight, and freeze can release through the supported introduction of new patterns of movement and through the unwinding of the old. Attunement to our inner world of senses and sensations can be amplified as we move. This awakens our sensitivity and thus our connection to all of life. Our emotions can be experienced and expressed as constrictive patterns thaw and life force is liberated. And as we move our bodies in uncharted non-linear patterns, new neural pathways in the brain are developed. In fact, dancing can actually be a natural antidepressant. It supports the release of endorphins from the brain into the bloodstream. This, in turn, produces a state of euphoria that can sometimes linger for hours and even days at a time.

Thus, as we move our bodies, we can literally open our hearts and liberate our minds. But that is not all. Dancing with a partner or in community is a way for people to meet their natural human need for positive social interaction. Imagine being in a room of other seniors who are not concerned about how they look, but rather are finding pleasure in moving to the music. Or, imagine the fun of holding hands with a friend, together gliding across the floor, your feet syncopated together in the beat. Whether whirling in a circle with dozens of others, or in a socially acceptable embrace while moving with one other, the eye to eye, heart to heart, and hand to hand human connection that happens when two or more are moving together is profoundly nurturing. A community that moves together provides the foundation for its people to both ground and to soar.

Dancing not only offers a doorway to connect with oneself and with others, but it can inspire powerful communion with something greater than us. For many, dancing is literally a spiritual experience. Dancing can be a portal to both the most sacred parts of our individual beings and to the Divine. As we ground our bodies, open our hearts, and expand our minds, the images rising up from our souls can become more visible. We can access the deeper myths guiding our unique journeys in life. Simultaneously, dance can also be a vehicle for communion with a vast transpersonal place that knows cosmic truths beyond one's personal story.

This universal portal to the sacred is a gift when our lives seem to make no sense, when pain is coursing through our bodies, when our hearts ache, or when we feel as if we are going out of our minds. Dance is a healing resource. So, when the day seems long or the grief seems bottomless, why not turn on some music and allow yourself to be moved out of inertia into action, out of isolation into connection, out of loss into love.

There are many wonderful ways to find one's way home through dance. Check out the internet or newspaper for weekly dance classes, special movement events, or gifted teachers offering workshops in your area. Try anything that calls to you. Trust your instincts about where you belong. Listen to your body about what feels just right and what does not. If you find a class too rigorous, tone it down for yourself. If you need more guidance than a teacher is offering, ask for it. If you love a class, return to it again and again. If you do not love it, skip it. Authenticity is the sexiest dance around, regardless of our age or physical prowess. And if an inspired class or moving service is not easily accessed in your area, your living room is a great place to begin.

What music moves you? From classical to world beat, there are endless sounds and rhythms that may just get you out of your seat and into the groove. New technologies make it simple to download music from every genre and diverse cultures around the world. Notice … Do you like smooth and melodic sounds? Or, do you prefer a bit of a hard and faster beat? What kinds of voices move you? Some music will remind you of days gone by. Allow yourself to dance to the oldies from your adolescence. When images surface of loved ones or funky events, let them wash through you. Keep on dancing. Other music will uplift you, reminding you of the vast universe that we are all a part of. Expand into that by allowing your body to breathe and be free.

If you are not so sure how to get moving, notice where you are already in motion and build on that. Follow the shaking out of your limbs after a shower, letting your whole body release. See if your knees can find a repetitive pattern that catalyzes your feet, hips, and spine to get into the action. It does not have to be about form and routines, although for some that is super engaging. For others, simply allowing the life force to flow through us in organic patterns is the natural high. Experiment. Try repeating the same movements to different kinds of music. Allow your emotions to lead you. Dance your fears, your anger, your grief, and your joy. See what emerges. Dance can be done free form, with or without music. Dance like water, earth, fire, air. Dance like the young child across the street or like the hawk flying overhead. Let all of life inspire your gestures. Even if you get bored, stay with it. Just beyond the resistance, there is a vast open landscape that we all long to be in. By putting the body into motion, healing happens. Our inherent intelligence comes into play. Our perspectives change. Our compassion for what is awakens. Beneath the stories we tell ourselves about our lives, there is a landscape of intelligence that both supports the development of our stories and liberates us from them.

The beauty of dance is that it can spontaneously be incorporated into one's life in a variety of ways, in a class or even alone in one's bathroom. Dance is an inexpensive, always accessible way of being with oneself, each other, and the Divine. In fact, a twenty-one year long Einstein Aging Study, completed in 2001, found that dancing is the best physical activity to help prevent dementia when compared to eleven other activities including team sports, swimming, and bicycling. The study (summarized in an article that appeared in the *New England Journal of Medicine* in 2003) indicates that frequent dancing can preventatively slow down cognitive decline. So let's get moving!

Whether we are struggling with our own health or tending to the needs of someone else, taking a break to breathe and reboot is key to the overall well-being of everyone. And if we want to release tension, pump our hearts, or free our minds while doing our daily prayers, dance guarantees to be a pleasurable path forward. It is a sure-fire way to get us out of our minds before we go out of our minds.

* * *

Melissa Michaels, EdD, is a registered Somatic Movement Educator and Therapist (ISMETA), the Founder and Director of Surfing The Creative® International Youth Rites of Passage Programs, Wild Life Productions, and Golden Bridge, a not-for-profit organization dedicated to improving and empowering the lives of young people through dance-based rites of passage programming. Building community through dance from conception through old age has been at the root of her work for decades. You can reach her at <u>office@bdanced.com</u>.

Music that will get you up on the floor

Dance Pop Songs

- James Brown - *Get Up (I Feel Like Being A) Sex Machine*
- Donna Summer - *Hot Stuff*
- Michael Jackson – *Thriller*
- B-52s - *Love Shack*
- Abba - *Dancing Queen*
- The Weather Girls - *It's Raining Men*
- The Bee Gees - *Stayin' Alive*
- Mariah Carey - *Fantasy*
- Whitney Houston - *I Wanna Dance With Somebody*
- Aretha Franklin - *Respect*

Big Band Songs

- Duke Ellington - *Take the "A" Train*
- Duke Ellington - *It Don't Mean a Thing*
- Glenn Miller - *Chattanooga Choo-Choo*
- Glenn Miller - *In the Mood*
- Glenn Miller - *Midnight Serenade*
- Benny Goodman - *Stompin' at the Savoy*
- Benny Goodman - *Sing, Sing, Sing*

- Erskine Hawkins - *Tuxedo Junction*
- Tommy Dorsey - *Song of India*
- Cole Porter (popularized by Artie Shaw) - *Begin the Beguine*

Salsa Music

- Oscar D'Leon - *Lloraras*
- Willie Colon - *Ojos*
- Fruko U Sus Tesos - *El Preso*
- India - *Vivir Lo Nuestro*
- Gambino Pampini - *Ave Maria Lola*
- Sonora Carruseles - *Micaela*
- Sonora Carruseles - *La Comay*
- Yuri Buenaventura - *Salsa*
- Joe Arroyo - *Rebelion*
- Marc Antony – *Vivir Mi Vida*

The Window

By **Barbra Cohn**

I'm coming home after dancing salsa. You're looking out your bedroom window, watching for me, waiting for me to drive into the driveway, wondering where I am and when I'll get home. You've probably been glued to the TV all evening, at least as long as your action-packed shows were on.

It's late. I'm late. I had an exhilarating time dancing with "my boys," as I call them; the salsa group I progress through, as they take turns twirling me and twisting my arms into moves called the hammerlock, sombrero, and arm loop. I don't ever want to stop. I don't want to come home to you. You, who have turned into my child, morphed in front of my eyes these past few years into a boy who needs help getting his pajamas on and one last drink of water.

The other night driving home in the dark I looked up at what used to be your window when you lived in the northeast bedroom on the third floor — before you moved to a memory care home. I recreated your watch-ful, bewildered look in my mind's eye, feeling your angst, feeling your trepidation, hearing your thoughts zigzag in your head, "Where is she? Where is Barbra? I don't like being here alone. I'm tired. I want to go to sleep."

Your fingerprints are still on the window you peered through. They remain a roadmap to your wondering, "Where is she? Why isn't she home?" They are the last bit of evidence of your existence on this earth. The rest of you is underground.

I caress the glass with my hands, tracing the tiny lines of your thumb, your index finger and ring finger. I gaze through them into the dark, watching for the ghost of me driving into the driveway late at night.

I place my feet on the carpet where you stood blowing smoke from the glass pipe filled with pot that helped you laugh and reach that place in yourself that used to be naturally relaxed.

Then, with one final intention I dip a sponge in water. Saturate it and squeeze out drops of water before I wipe the window clean. I start from the top moving horizontally like a skier traversing the slope. From right to left and left to right I move the sponge deliberately. I change direction and move it vertically to wash away your handprint, the curlicues and whorls of your fingers until the glass is transparent and void of your cells, and the last bit of physical evidence that you lived in this house and on this earth.

* * *

References

Ambrose, Anne F., Herman Buschke, Carol A. Derby, Charles B. Hall, Mindy J. Katz, Gail Kuslansky, Richard B. Lipton, Martin Sliwinski, and Joe Verghese. 2003. "Leisure Activities and the Risk of Dementia in the Elderly." *The New England Journal of Medicine*. 348: 2508-2516.

23

Drumming

The simple act of drumming can enable a non-verbal person with dementia to communicate—albeit temporarily—with loved ones. The physical, mental, and emotional benefits of drumming are discussed in this chapter, as well as information on how you can find a drumming circle in your location.

"Group drumming tunes our biology, orchestrates our immunity, and enables healing to begin."
– Barry Bittman, MD.

Drumming for Caregivers and Alzheimer's and Dementia Patients

By **John K. Galm**, PhD

The magic pulsations of drumbeats have been used throughout the ages in many cultures for healing and building cultural values. These drumbeats have seldom been used with Alzheimer's patients and their caregivers. The following is a description and commentary on my experience using the pulsing rhythm of drumming with a group of dementia patients and their caregivers.

The process

Eight people with various stages of Alzheimer's disease and their caregivers enter a comfortable room with reduced lighting. The afternoon light shines on a circle of chairs with a large Native American powwow drum, horizontally placed in the center. After a brief social period, I describe the drumming technique as non-invasive. The participants have the option of participating or observing, and everyone agrees. We enter a short period of silence and then I distribute percussion instruments: small drums with beaters, hand shakers, rattles, claves or rhythm sticks, and other easy-to-play instruments.

I softly play the large Native American drum, with a steady pulse of about sixty beats per minute. (The normal heart rate for adults ranges from sixty to one hundred beats per minute.) The participants can join the pulsing with their hand-held instruments or just listen. They enter the playing or withdraw as they wish. The pulse fluctuates with a slight increase in speed and gets louder or softer as the dynamic flow of the group changes during the natural unfolding of the drumming. I am the only one that plays the large drum in the center so that I can guide the process.

After forty-five minutes, the group feels the drumming fade and becomes silent. The percussion instruments are placed aside and the silence is observed until one of the people with Alzheimer's communicates through speech or gesture. This beautiful period allows most of the caregivers to converse with their loved-ones. Some people are not able to respond, but they seem rested and at ease. This communication period lasts for minutes, hours, or in some cases the entire afternoon. Then the veils of Alzheimer's descend once again.

What happens and why

No medical research has been conducted on this process to determine why drumming allows the Alzheimer's condition to be temporarily lifted. Music Therapy studies suggest that perhaps the normal pulsations of the body are strengthened or recomposed during drumming. Some practitioners of Chinese Medicine can determine the pulse rate of many bodily functions, such as heartbeat, respiration, liver, stomach, etc. and through acupuncture or herbs can restore the pulse rate to a normal condition. Some drumming therapies can affect the same. Along with reprogramming and stimulating the bodily pulses, the aspect of drumming in a community has a therapeutic effect of unification and well-being. Many drum circles that I have led or participated in have resulted in a joyous occasion with the drummers feeling a communal spirit of elation.

Another aspect of this process is the concept of "entrainment," which is that situation where a more powerful rhythmic vibration can change the less powerful vibrations and synchronize their rhythms. The drumming usually lasts for at least twenty minutes to achieve this effect. Through sound and pulsation, it is possible to change the rhythms of heartbeats, respiration, and brainwaves, etc. This concept is very strong in West African drumming where the drumming entrains the community by unifying and strengthening various life rituals and the culture itself.

When a person creates a sound with a physical motion, as opposed to just listening to the sound, the effect allows the body to absorb the pulsing. Brain research has identified that area where sound is translated into motor activity. Unfortunately, this tradition of movement and music has been almost lost in Western culture today. Many other cultures continue this unification of dance and music to the extent that they have no term for music or dance separately in their languages.

Blessings

Caregivers have given many accounts of how drumming allows a communication to take place in a unique situation. Here are some of the reactions that I've heard:

"I never thought I would be able to reach him again."

"What joy to feel her respond to me."

"The times of frustration and loneliness vanished in these moments."

The time and space is shared in the power of a transforming and healing atmosphere, and the participants also feel the joy of the communal participation. I hope that this non-invasive process of communal drumming will become a popular therapy for working with caregivers and their care partners who have Alzheimer's disease and dementia.

* * *

Dr. **John K. Galm** *is Professor Emeritus in Ethnomusicology at the University of Colorado. He has studied traditional music in Bali, India, Senegal, Turkey, and Morocco, and has presented concerts and workshops in the United States, Canada, Europe, West Africa, Turkey, and Brazil. He has contributed many articles to the international journal "Percussive Notes" and to "The Encyclopedia of Percussion Instruments." Since retirement, he has given lectures and concerts and conducted Sound Healing Workshops with Jonathan Goldman and Vickie Dodd.*

Drumming for care partners

I attended a drumming circle with Morris at the memory care home where he lived. The leader, John Crowder JD, trained directly with neurologist Barry Bittman, MD, and Christine Stevens, MSW- MT-BC, through the Health Rhythms™ program.

"You know, we all have a drum right here," Crowder said, pointing to his heart. At least half of the members of the group understood exactly what he meant, as they shook their gourds to the rhythm of his drum.

But when Crowder handed out conga drums and other hand-held instruments, that's when the fun really began. At the end of each rhythmic song, one patient would tell about his adventures in the military. And he didn't miss a beat. More than once he broke into song, "Over hill, over dale, we would chase all kinds of tail."

A woman talked about how her father and brother were drummers. Even though she insisted that she had never drummed, she apparently had learned by listening and watching because she was quite adept at following Crowder's rhythms and creating rhythms for the rest of the group to follow. Throughout the forty-five minute session several people broke into song, which Crowder used to simultaneously lead the group in singing and playing. Several times he had the group mimic his rhythm. Overall, it was a calming, enjoyable experience for everyone.

Drumming for caregivers

Drumming is equally beneficial for caregivers. Dr. Bittman conducted landmark research published in *Alternative Therapies in Health and Medicine*, 2001, which showed that group drumming therapy releases stress and increases the disease-fighting activity of white blood cells.

Another study showed that long-term care workers experienced less burnout, stress, and mood disturbances when they participated in a six-week program of recreational music-making, defined as distinct from "regular" music making, as its purpose is the enjoyment and well-being of the participants, not an artistic or aesthetic outcome that requires talent or training.

Drumming circles are a fun and healthy way to connect with your care partner. To find a drumming circle in your location, visit the USA Drum Circle Finder website: drumcircles.net/circlelist.html. Or buy a couple of drums and create your own drumming experience. Visit the Drum Circles Network website for information on drums, DVDs, and other information to help you get started. drumcircles.net

* * *

References

Bittman, Barry B., Karl T. Bruhn. Christine Stevens, James Westengard, and Paul Umbach. 2003. "Recreational Music-Making: A Cost-Effective Group Interdisciplinary Strategy for Reducing Burnout and Improving Mood States in Long-Term Care Workers." *Advances in Mind-Body Medicine*. 19: 4-15.

Bittman, Barry B., Lee S Berk, David Felten, James Westengard, Carfl Simonton, James Pappas, and Melissa Ninehouser. 2001. "Composite Effects of Group Drumming Music Therapy on Modulation of Neuro-endocrine-Immune Parameters in Normal Subject." *Alternative Therapies in Health and Medicine*. 7(1): 38-47.

Diallo, Yaya and Mitch Hall. *The Healing Drum: African Wisdom Teachings*. (Rochester, VT: Destiny Books, 1989).

Diamond, John. *The Way of the Pulse; Drumming with Spirit*. (Bloomingdale, IL: Enhancement Books, 1999).

Friedman, Robert Lawrence. *The Healing Power of the Drum*. (Tempe, AZ: White Cliffs Media Co, 2000).

Goldman, Jonathan. *Healing Sounds: The Power of Harmonics*. (Rochester, VT: Healing Arts Press, 1992).

Levitin, Daniel. *This is Your Brain on Music*. (New York, NY: Penguin Group 2006).

Stevens, Christine. *The Art and Heart of Drum Circles*. (Milwaukee, WI: Hal Leonard Corporation, 2003).

24

Exercise

We've all heard how important exercise is to our health and well-being. But now researchers have proof that exercise is vital to protecting the body from stress, depression, and anxiety. In this chapter you'll hear the scientific explanation from Monika Fleshner, PhD, and how the simple routine of walking can make a huge difference in your vitality, health, and mood.

"If you are in a bad mood go for a walk. If you are still in a bad mood go for another walk." – Hippocrates

The Physiology of Stress

Statistics show that the stress of caregiving can result in chronic disease for the caregiver and take as many as ten years off one's life. First described by Walter Cannon in the 1920s, the fight-or-flight response, also called the acute stress response, kicks in when we are presented with danger or an emergency. Our brains react quickly to keep us safe by preparing the body for action. Hunters who were responsible for killing game to provide food for their tribe and the animals being hunted experienced the fight-or-flight response on a regular basis. Unfortunately today, because of the stressful world we live in, the fight-or-flight response is more commonly triggered by psychological threats than physical ones, such as an argument with a spouse, demanding bosses, out-of-control drivers, road rage, etc.

In the physiological response to stress, pupils dilate to sharpen vision, and heart rate and blood pressure increase to accelerate the delivery of oxygen to fuel muscles and critical organs. Blood flow is diverted from non-critical areas, such as the gastrointestinal tract, to the critical areas, such as the heart, skeletal muscles, and liver.

The liver releases glucose and fatty acids into the bloodstream. Glucose is for immediate energy; fat is needed when the fight-or-flight response lasts longer than expected. Bronchial tubes dilate to maximize the exchange of oxygen and carbon dioxide.

When the body is in a constant state of "emergency alert" due to chronic stress such as caregiving, the adrenal glands—the small walnut shaped glands that sit on top of your kidneys—get "stuck" in the on position. When this happens, the whole system goes into chronic fight-or-flight. Glucose that is dumped into your bloodstream goes unused, so your body has to produce an enormous amount of insulin to handle it. Eventually, this can result in hypoglycemia or diabetes. Fat that is dumped into your blood also goes unused, so it clogs your arteries, leading to cardiovascular disease. If you drink three or more cups of coffee every day, the stress hormone cortisol becomes elevated, which can set you up for countless health problems, including poor quality of sleep, impaired immunity, and age-related deterioration.

Adrenal exhaustion

The adrenal glands produce or contribute to the production of about one hundred and fifty hormones. When they are repeatedly and intensely activated to make hormones, the adrenals can become exhausted. Once the adrenal buffer is gone, you become a prime candidate for asthma, allergies, fibromyalgia, chronic fatigue syndrome, autoimmune disorders, hypoglycemia, and more.

Alcohol, caffeine, sugar, and salt put added stress on the adrenals. Stimulants such as caffeine increase the effects of your body's own stimulating neurotransmitters, norepinephrine and dopamine, which are similar to adrenaline in their effects. Caffeine and these natural stimulants provide short-term energy, focus, and even a lifted mood. But in the long term, caffeine depletes your stores of norepinephrine and dopamine, leaving you more tired, sluggish, and down than you were before you developed a caffeine habit.

Adequate sleep, a nutritious diet, and all the modalities in this book can definitely help manage stress. Dr. Monika Fleshner, PhD, professor in the Department of Integrative Physiology and the Center for Neuroscience at the University of Colorado, says there is something extra special about exercise versus other modalities for reducing stress, which she explains in her article, "Exercise and Stress Robustness: Benefits for Mental and Physical Health."

Exercise raises your metabolism, enabling your body to burn calories more efficiently and at a faster rate. But exercise is much more than a great way to control your weight. It is a mood, mind, and memory enhancer. Lack of exercise lowers metabolic efficiency and without circulatory stimulation, the body's natural circulatory and cleansing systems are weakened.

Cardiovascular exercise stimulates the entire body, encouraging lymphatic drainage, healthy lung capacity, heart strength, and optimum circulation. Exercise also changes the brain in ways that protect memory and thinking skills. In a study at the University of British Columbia, researchers found that regular aerobic exercise appears to boost the size of the hippocampus, the brain area involved in verbal memory and learning. Perhaps most importantly for caregivers, exercise reduces stress.

Exercise and Stress Robustness: Benefits for Mental and Physical Health

By **Monika Fleshner**, PhD

Stress is a part of life, and it can be a friend or foe. Good stress acts as a motivator. For instance, deadlines at work or school provide the incentive to complete a task. Stress is our response to a particular event. If we are caring for someone 24/7 the caregiving is the stressor, and how we respond to the task is the stress.

When we are in an acute state of stress, the body responds by increasing concentrations of powerful pro and anti-inflammatory proteins that can help get cells of the immune system ready to respond to infection or injury. A major contributor stimulating this whole body state of immune preparation is the sympathetic nervous system. When the sympathetic nervous system is activated, the nerves that innervate all tissues in the body release norepinephrine into many tissues in the body and into the blood. For example, sympathetic nervous system activation increases heart rate, enlarges pupils, and stimulates sweating, as described in the fight-or-flight response. All this helps us fight or flee. It's a fast on/

off response. When we can't turn the stress off, the powerful stress hormones become damaging to the organs and rest of the body.

If stressors are severe, uncontrollable, repeated, and chronic, and/or if we are vulnerable to other health problems, we can suffer both mental and physical problems. What can we do to protect ourselves since life's stressors are unavoidable? Maintaining a physically active lifestyle might be one solution.

How does exercise counteract stress?

Based on the research that my colleagues and I have done in the past thirteen years, we know that regular physical activity promotes stress robustness (resistance to stress) and changes the way the brain and body respond to stressors. Regular physical activity is good for your body and mind. In fact, in 2007 The American College of Sports Medicine (ACSM) and the American Medical Association (AMA) launched Exercise is Medicine™, a program designed to encourage Americans to incorporate physical activity and exercise into their daily routine. Exercise is Medicine™ even calls on doctors to prescribe exercise to their patients.

If you are highly conditioned from a regular exercise routine, then you can respond better psychologically and physically. We can directly measure the effect that stressors and stress have on laboratory animals in a controlled environment and then predict parallel outcomes for humans. Excessive, acute, and chronic activation of the stress response is associated with an increased risk of harmful physical and mental consequences. Many factors such as age, gender, and genetics will play a part in the impact of stress on one's physical and mental state.

Whether you feel that you have control or not, controllability — as in the number of minutes you exercise each day or the amount of nutritious foods you eat as opposed to junk foods — helps mitigate the negative effects of stress. A person's physical activity status (sedentary versus active) has a big impact. Sedentary individuals are more vulnerable to cardiovascular disease, diabetes, anxiety, depression, obesity, and other health conditions. On the other hand, physically active individuals are "stress robust." They demonstrate both stress resistance and stress resilience. Stress resistance delays the tipping point. It increases the intensity or duration of stress or exposure needed to move from positive to negative consequences of stress. When organisms and humans have stress resilience, they are capable of bouncing back quickly after crossing the tipping point.

There is something extra special about exercise versus other modalities for reducing stress. The chemicals in the brain of someone who exercises stimulate normal growth and survival hormones, as well as an active immune response to inflammation. Exercise seems to buffer many of the deleterious consequences of stress.

Activity supports a better immune response

Stress in sedentary rats can alter the development and healing time of inflammation caused by bacterial infection. In my laboratory test, results showed that when sedentary rats infected with E. coli bacteria were exposed to an acute stressor their inflammation resolved faster than in the non-stressed rats infected with the bacteria.

In recent years, inflammation has been linked to numerous degenerative diseases. But inflammation, like stress, can be a good thing. A cut on the hand becomes inflamed because an increase of white blood cells and antigens rush to the area in order to heal it.

In comparison to the stressed sedentary rats, stressed rats that had been regularly running on a wheel and were then infected showed an increase in bacteria-attacking white blood cells migrating to the infection site, causing the healing time to speed up by three to four days faster than the sedentary stressed rat.

An analogy might be a sedentary person on a challenging mountain hike cutting his hand on a sharp rock and introducing bacteria into the wound. That person's body probably would not be able to 'clean up' the infection site as quickly or efficiently as an experienced, active mountain climber's body.

The converse is also true. When an organism is overwhelmed with stress, there might be an overproduction of too many cytokines, a class of proteins that are linked to inflammation or swelling of body tissues. These proteins typically emerge when the body is fighting off a disease. In one of our laboratory tests, we found that rats that were exposed to an acute severe stressor had elevated concentrations of the inflammatory proteins. The important things to remember are that stress modulates our immune response and that physical activity prevents the negative impacts and promotes the beneficial consequences of stress on immunity.

Exercise reduces depression and anxiety

In numerous studies, we found that laboratory rats that run on a wheel for up to six weeks exhibit less anxiety and behavioral depression when exposed to a stressor compared to sedentary animals. This work is important because it allows us to measure specific changes in neural circuits of the brain that function to promote stress resistance. We have revealed several mechanisms by which exercise confers protection against stress-induced behaviors and they include changes in brain serotonin circuits, brain inflammatory molecules and genes involved with diurnal rhythms.

Additionally, the exercised rats showed overall health improvements in many areas:

- Decrease in body weight gain
- Improved visceral fitness (less abdominal fat)
- Decrease in triglycerides and hypertension
- Increase in lipid metabolism
- Increase in HDL/LDL ratio
- Increased red blood count hemoglobin capacity
- Improved endurance
- Increased social exploration

Physical exercise can provide you with the ability to endure the consequences of chronic stress without suffering long-term negative mental and physical health consequences. But it's difficult. For optimal protection it's important to sustain a regular exercise program, which could be as simple as walking thirty minutes every day. Maintaining a regular schedule is important, including the length of time you exercise and the time of day. This is probably important because one change that predicts long-term negative consequences of stress is disrupted diurnal rhythms.

Every cell in our brain and body functions in a diurnally oscillating way. We evolved on a planet that rotates on its axis and produces repeated cycles of light and dark. Exposure to chronic and repeated stressors flattens our rhythms and flattened rhythms are associated with negative mental and physical health. It seems feasible that regular exercise, especially at specific times of day, could protect our diurnal rhythms from stressor-evoked disruptions.

Do we have to exercise every day to have these protective effects? Based on our study of rats, we know that we can slack off for a couple of weeks before losing the protective effect that exercise provides against uncontrollable stress.

Life is filled with emotional and physical challenges or stressors. Our physiology has evolved to respond to these challenges, and in fact, elevate our level of mental and physical function to rise to the challenge and succeed! If those challenges persist, and we are not physically fit, not healthy, or older, we can suffer the negative consequences of exposure to life's challenges. Regular physical activity helps promote stress resistance so we can endure challenges or stressors longer and promotes stress resilience so we can recover after suffering negative health consequences.

* * *

Monika Fleshner, PhD is a professor in the Department of Integrative Physiology and the Center for Neuroscience at the University of Colorado, president of The International Society of Exercise and Immunology, and author of nearly one hundred and forty papers in a variety of scientific journals. Her research program is focused on understanding the impact of acute and chronic stress on behavior, neural, hormonal, and immunological function and on the physiological benefits of exercise and how it counteracts stress. E-mail: monika.fleshner@colorado.edu

* * *

How Exercise Helped Us Cope With Alzheimer's

By **Mattye Pollard-Cole**

I think I was able to cope pretty well with my husband Cliff's Alzheimer's because I exercised almost daily. If nothing else, I went for an early morning walk. It was a good time to be alone with my thoughts while I enjoyed being outdoors or golfing with friends or working out at our health club. Exercise enabled me to stay fairly positive. Without it, I would have been depressed and probably on an antidepressant.

Exercise is also great for the person with Alzheimer's. Even though Cliff lost many cognitive skills and the ability to read and write, he was strong and was able to continue physical activities for a long time. This helped his mood and also helped him to sleep through the night. Cliff had been a good athlete all his life, excelling in kayaking, bicycling, swimming, and skiing, so it was natural for him to continue exercising after he became ill.

When Cliff was first diagnosed at age fifty-five, we continued to go on long bike rides together. However, there were two scary incidents. First, in June 2006 (two years after his diagnosis) Cliff and I were riding together and Cliff got separated from me on the way home. He was lost for about four hours, but finally called home from an office building more than five miles from where he got lost. After that, I got him a Project Lifesaver wristband.* Then in June 2007, we were riding and Cliff fell and injured his shoulder, for which he needed surgery. At that point, he was having trouble with balance and making decisions on the road, and it became too difficult for him to ride outside any longer.

From 2007 to December 2009, Cliff and I took Spinning classes at our health club, and we went for long walks. Cliff also swam laps about once a week. Although he was able to swim quite well, I had to hire a caregiver to supervise him in the pool because he was unable to stay in his lane. Cliff exercised at least three times a week until late 2009.

I maintained Cliff's membership at the club through December 2009. By the end of that year it was very difficult to get him to go to the club, but we continued to take walks together. I placed him at The Court, a memory care home, in February 2010 and when I visited him there we went for short walks outside. As time progressed, Cliff had more and more difficulty walking. By the time he died in March 2011, it would take two of us to get him up to walk, and then only with difficulty. Cliff was close to being wheelchair-bound by the time he died. I'm sure exercise helped him to stay healthier and enjoy a fuller life in his last years.

* * *

*Project Lifesaver provides police, fire/rescue, and other first responders with a comprehensive program including equipment and training to quickly locate and rescue "at risk" individuals with cognitive disorders who are at constant risk to the life threatening behavior of wandering, including those with Alzheimer's disease, Autism, and Down's Syndrome. If an enrolled client goes missing, the caregiver notifies their local Project Lifesaver agency, and a trained emergency team responds to the wanderer's area. Recovery times for PLI clients average thirty minutes — ninety-five percent less time than standard operations. www.projectlifesaver. org/about-us.

* * *

Implementing a fun exercise program

Most people exercise to burn calories, but the harder we exercise, the more endorphins we produce. The stress of exercise triggers the release of the "feel good" chemicals from the brain into the bloodstream. The endorphins then attach to nerve receptors, there is relief from pain, and the bonus is an "exercise high," or feeling of euphoria. It generally takes at least thirty minutes of continuous aerobic exercise before endorphins kick in, so it is advisable to stick with it!

Other caregivers I've talked with claim that exercise is the main thing that kept them sane throughout the caregiving process. So make it a priority to get at least thirty minutes a day. It's not necessary to go to a gym or buy fancy equipment. Take a walk, and if you need a motivator, ask a neighbor or friend to do a regular walk. Here are some other ideas:

- Buy a new pair of athletic shoes that do an excellent job of supporting feet and ankles.

- Go for a walk! Or get into a routine. It it's been a while since you've worked your muscles, start out with an easy walk for twenty minutes, three times a week. Gradually increase the time, frequency, and tempo until you're up to at least thirty minutes, three to five days a week.

- Dance the night away. Put on your favorite music and dance in your living room, alone or with your care partner. Or rent a dance instruction DVD and boogie! Chances are no one will be watching. (Read chapter 13, *Dance as Exercise* for more information.)

- Hike into the wild blue yonder. Whether you live in the southwest desert, southeast wetlands, or northeast mountains, there's bound to be a hiking trail nearby. Put on a pair of sturdy shoes, sun block, and get out and enjoy nature. It'll clear your mind and boost your energy.

* * *

References

Adler, Nancy E., Elizabeth H. Blackburn, Richard M. Cawthon, Firadaus S. Dhabhar, Elissa S. Epel, Jue Kin, and Jason D. Morrow. 2004. "Accelerated telomere shortening in response to life stress." *Proceedings of the National Academy of Sciences of the United States of America.* 101(4): 17312-5.

Beninson, Lida, Monika Fleshner, Benjamin N. Greenwood, Lucas Mahaffey, Thomas Maslanik, and Kate Tannura. 2012. "The inflammasome and danger associated molecular patterns (DAMPs) are implicated in cytokine and chemokine responses following stressor exposure." *Brain Behavior and Immunity.* 54-62.

Bolandzadeh, Niousha, Lisanne ten Brinke, Jennifer C Davis, Chun Liang Hsu, Karim M Khan, and Lindsay S Nagamatsu. 2013. "Aerobic exercise increases hippocampal volume in older women with probable mild cognitive impairment: a 6-month randomized controlled trial." *British Journal of Sports Medicine.* 49(4): 248-254.

Cannon, Walter B. *Bodily Changes in Pain Hunger Fear And Rage.* (Charleston, SC: Nabu Press, 1929).

Day, Heidi E.W., Monika Fleshner, Benjamin N. Greenwood, Alice B. Loughridge, and Matthew B. McQueen. 2013. "Microarray analyses reveal novel targets of exercise-induced stress resistance in the dorsal raphe nucleus." *Frontiers in Behavioral Neuroscience.*

Emmons, Henry and Rachel Kranz. *The Chemistry of Joy: A Three-Step Program for Overcoming Depression Through Western Science and Eastern Wisdom.* (New York, NY: Simon & Schuster, Inc., 2006).

Fleshner, Monika, Benjamin N. Greenwood, Alice B. Loughridge, N. Sadaoui, and J.P. Christianson. 2012. "The protective effects of voluntary exercise against the behavioral consequences of uncontrollable stress persist despite an increase in anxiety following forced cessation of exercise." *Behavior Brain Research.* 233(2): 314-21.

Fleshner, Monika, Benjamin N. Greenwood, and Robert S. Thompson. 2013. "Impact of physical activity on diurnal rhythms: A potential mechanism for exercise-induced stress resistance and stress resilience." In *Routledge Handbook of Physical Activity and Mental Health.* 316-28.

Fleshner, Monika, Paul v. Strong, and Robert S. Thompson. 2012. "Physiological consequences of repeated exposure to conditioned fear." *Behavioral Sciences.* 2(2): 57-78.

25

Horticultural Therapy (Gardening)

All you need is a bag of soil, pair of gloves, a planter, trowel, and plants to evoke memories and to create an uplifting spiritual, sensory experience for a care partner with dementia. This chapter offers the information you need to get started, including a recommended list of plants and materials.

"Many things grow in the garden that were never sown there."
– Thomas Fuller, *Gnomologia*

By **Pam Catlin**

There has likely never been a time when a connection between people and plants did not exist. Plant life does make a difference in reducing stress. Studies have shown that you can reduce your blood pressure by simply looking at plants. Outdoor and indoor plantings help to create an inviting, calming, and often familiar atmosphere. For many elders, gardening has been a part of life, especially early life. Long-term memories of Grandma's herb garden or of helping Father harvest vegetables will often bring back a sense of peace and happiness.

The garden provides a place for releasing tension through walking, weeding, and digging. For caregivers, a simple patio garden can provide a place of peaceful refuge for themselves, as well as a place to connect more deeply with their loved one. Plants provide an opportunity for communicating in a world where the old ways of sharing no longer suffice.

Improving physical health

An obvious physical benefit of gardening is simply getting fresh air and sunshine. Working with plants can also provide a way to maintain or improve motor skills. Some exercises that seemed impossible in the sterile environment of the physical therapy room are done without hesitation as one reaches to harvest a tomato or plant a flower. An individual is able to develop stamina for standing with the support of a raised bed garden. And folks with arthritic fingers can usually use lightweight tools with foam-covered handles. Whether indoors or out, tasks such as watering, grooming, mixing soil, or arranging flowers naturally encourage the use of fine and gross motor skills.

Improving mental health

At this stage of life with memory loss, many individuals have lost the responsibility that was once a part of their daily routine. Lacking a sense of purpose and importance can dramatically affect one's sense of self-esteem and ability to thrive. In caring for plants, there are tasks that are appropriate for almost any level of functioning, thus providing purposeful activity in the midst of most stages of memory loss. For those who are receiving so much care, the plants provide an opportunity to give care. Another aspect of building self-esteem is the ability to give to others. Everyone enjoys receiving, yet giving is just as valuable and more difficult for the person with advanced cognitive issues. Plant activities can provide the gardener with lovely items, such as potted plants or flower arrangements, to share with family and friends.

Supporting spiritual growth

The spiritual benefits of nature are undeniable. The miracle of new life each time a seed germinates, a cutting takes root, or spring leaves burst forth is a constant reminder of our connection to all life. As one gardener said on a beautiful day outdoors, "We are one with all." The cycle of life, as demonstrated by plants, can be a comfort when considering one's own life journey. Seasons in a garden all have their own unique beauty and purpose, as do the seasons of our own lives. Television, magazines, and movies fail to share this message, yet the garden does it so reliably. Taking time to just "be" in the garden, observing, listening, and breathing it all in, supports the deeper recognition of a spiritual connection.

Promoting sensory stimulation

The plant world offers an almost endless source of sensory stimulation. A well-planned garden can provide an awakening for all the senses. When gardening with individuals who have severe cognitive impairment, it is essential to have only non-toxic plants in the garden and to avoid plants with sharp thorns or spines that could tear the skin. If you are in doubt, research the plant to ensure its safety.

Throughout the ages people have connected over food, and the garden setting provides an abundance of taste experiences through edible flowers, herbs, and vegetables. Not all non-poisonous flowers are tasty or have a pleasing texture, however. Some tried and true edible flowers are nasturtiums, lavender, day lilies, roses, tulips, pansies, and violas. The flowers can be used in salads, baking, decorating cakes, and so much more. In caring for these flowers, make sure you avoid chemical pesticides.

Herbs and vegetables are a great addition to a garden and they provide another taste experience. Basil, chives, mint, oregano, parsley, and rosemary are all easy-to-grow herbs. Some are even perennials that will come back each year. Enjoy these herbs by mixing them into plain yogurt or softened cream cheese to create an easy dip to spread on crackers and veggies. When you are selecting vegetable plants, keep in mind that plants in the solanaceous family (tomatoes and eggplant) have toxic foliage. Most gardeners love a beautiful, ripe tomato, so just be careful to supervise the planting and care of these plants.

People who have retained their olfactory senses will enjoy the fragrance of herbs when they run their hands over the herb plants. Sweet alyssum, heliotrope, pansies, and cosmos are particularly fragrant flowers. Scented geraniums, grown for their foliage and not their bloom, date back to Victorian times and are now available in most nurseries in a variety of fragrances, including citrus, chocolate, and rose.

When you select plants to stimulate the visual senses, it is important to remember that older eyes have an easier time seeing bright colors such as reds, pinks, and yellows than subtle, pastel colors or white. Don't forget interesting leaf patterns when you're looking for visual stimuli. You can find unusual leaf patterns and colors in coleus, Rex begonias, and some grasses, such as zebra grass.

Consider adding some auditory elements to the garden. Wind chimes near the patio door can assist in orienting an individual to the door's location. Grasses, trees, plants with seed pods, water features, and bird feeders can all add a variety of pleasant sounds to the garden.

As the other senses fade, tactile stimulation becomes an important part of the gardening experience. Selections that are surprisingly soft to the touch are dusty miller, African fountain grass, and lamb's ears. Smooth skinned succulents provide tactile interest and can be grown indoors and, weather permitting, outdoors. Placing plants with texture near the edges of containers or beds is an invitation for visitors to touch and feel, as they move through the outdoor space. Try running a fuzzy leaf across the cheek of a memory-impaired gardener who isn't responsive to the touch of a plant. The "apple" of the cheek is filled with tiny nerve endings that are often more receptive than the nerve endings in older fingers.

How to set up a therapy garden for your yard or porch

As the person with memory loss advances in his or her disease process, physical balance tends to become a challenge. An effective way to create a safe gardening experience is to elevate the growing areas either through raised beds or large pots. For those able to stand for short periods of time, a variety of planter heights would be ideal to support gardening while standing or sitting. The recommended dimensions for planter height is 2'-2 ½' for sitting, or 3'-3 ½' for standing. Acceptable dimensions for widths are 2' if accessible from only one side, or 4' if accessible from all sides. If the gardener has limited reach, avoid building materials such as bricks or block, since it would be difficult to reach the soil to plant. It's a good idea to measure what would be comfortable for the user before constructing the garden.

Growing in pots or raised beds requires good planting mixes (combination of peat moss, topsoil, and sand or perlite, or a good quality soil-less mix), regular fertilizing, and plants that are no taller than 3'. These days, many large pots are lightweight and easy to move and place prior to filling with soil mix. Pots can be placed on rolling saucers, provided the wheels have brakes, or on pavers to help raise them to an appropriate height.

The garden's walking surface should be relatively flat, smooth, well-draining, and uniform in appearance. As a person advances in memory loss, he or she will possibly become afraid of changes in pathway surfaces. For example, if the pathway from a cement patio to another area is made of decomposed granite, the person might be afraid to step past the edge of the patio. Consistency in texture and color will help to avoid this occurrence. When cement is used for patios and walkways, it is ideal to brush and tint the paving. Brushing provides a more non-slip surface, and tinting helps to diminish glare that is uncomfortable to most elders' eyes.

Lightweight hoses and long "water wands" or automatic irriga-tion make watering easier and safe. Don't forget to add a table and chairs for sitting and enjoying the beauty and bounty of the garden. More information on construction, soil mixes, feeding, watering, and tools can be found in books on raised bed and con-tainer gardening. An excellent book on gardening for people with disabilities is *The Enabling Garden: Creating Barrier-Free Gardens*, (1996) by Gene Rothert.

Successful plants

There are a number of tried and true plants that are safe for the garden. For cool weather gardening, calendulas, pansies/violas, and stock add bright color. Cool season vegetables include broccoli, cabbage, cauliflower, kale, lettuce, peas, radishes, and spinach. Coleus, impatiens, begonias, and mint are suitable for the warm season shade garden. Good plants for warm season sunny loca-tions are: Alyssum, dusty miller, geraniums, marigolds, purple cup flower, petunias, portulaca, snapdragons, zinnias, and most herbs other than mint, and most vegetables other than those men-tioned for cool season planting. Bush varieties of squashes and cucumbers are best suited for raised beds and pots, as are some varieties of tomatoes.

A piece of advice when creating a garden space is to start small. The primary purpose of this growing area is not food production. Its purpose is to provide peace of mind and an avenue of connection for you and your care partner. A garden that provides a balance of physical activity and just *being* in nature is a perfect addition to your overall care plan.

* * *

Pam Catlin *is a horticultural therapist, registered through the American Horticultural Therapy Association (AHTA). She has been working in the field of horticultural therapy (HT) since 1976. During that time, prior to moving to Prescott, Arizona, she developed HT programs in WA, OR, and IL and served as director of horticultural therapy services for Chicago Botanic Garden. Reach Pam at* pcatlin72@gmail.com*.*

26

Humor

Everyone loves to laugh. Learn how humor can help you get closer to your care partner, and be used as a tool to diffuse stress and anger and support health. You'll also learn ways to incorporate humor into your care giving.

"A day without laughter is a day wasted."
– Charlie Chaplin

You gotta have a sense of humor

Although I shed more tears in the years I took care of Morris than in all my previous years combined, I also had some good laughs. And while some might interpret laughing at what comes out of the mouth of a memory-impaired person as an insult, I think of it as a response to the absurdity of how the mind works in this complicated disease; that is, how rational thinking is replaced by haphazard, illogical thinking.

For example, before Morris began losing the ability to read he would join me in the morning ritual of reading the paper at the breakfast table. We would scan the paper and discuss interesting stories. One morning I read aloud a piece about a study in which a potential Alzheimer's drug was found to remove amyloid plaque from the brains of laboratory mice. Morris, who complained 365 days of the year—morning *and* evening—about taking his pills, looked up from the paper and said, "What? Now I have to take mice?"

When the stock show comes to Denver every January, the evening news typically features a related oddball story. One night, a young girl was shown with her prized hog named Cinderella, whom she was raising to sell for a profit. Morris looked up from his dinner plate and said, "What? They're going to sell Cinderella?" (He, of course, was referring to the fairytale Cinderella.)

When I handed him a sandwich to eat, he asked me what it was. I replied, "Chicken salad." He threw the sandwich across the table and exclaimed, "This chicken is dead!"

Sometimes I laughed uncontrollably when he came out with these nonsensical comments. And sometimes I wondered if the inflated laughter was just a way of releasing pent up stress and anxiety. Understanding the facts about what laughter does for the mind, body, and soul is the first step to making it a priority as a caregiver. Rather than turning to food, alcohol, or other types of self-destructive behavior to relieve stress, the experience of humor provides a sound and healthy alternative to *decrease stress and feel happy.*

Laughter yoga

When I was a child, my mother and I would sometimes go into the living room after dinner, lie on the carpeted floor, and just roll around and laugh. Today, people get paid to guide others in "laughter yoga." Laughter is naturally contagious, and there's nothing more fun than getting together with a group of people and laughing until your sides ache.

For information about Laughter Yoga, where to find a laughter event, and for Laughter Yoga products (DVD/s CD's and audio-video downloads) visit www.laughteryoga.org/english.

Humor as a Stress Diffuser and Health Promoter

By **Heather Hans**, LSW, MSW, CPIC, MSBA

Incorporating humor into day-to-day caregiving can help lighten the load and help caregivers to stay positive. Transitions can be challenging, and humor can keep the bond strong between the caregiver and the Alzheimer's patient, despite the changing relationship dynamic. Love is the core of any relationship and paves the path that two people share together on earth. Laughing at some of the absurdities presented by Alzheimer's disease can remind the caregiver of the sweet soul that is separate from the failing mind and body of the person they are caring for.

The health benefits of humor are vast. Four of the top physical health benefits are: increased immunity, decreased pain, muscle relaxation for up to forty-five minutes after laughing, and decreased risk of cardiovascular disease. A 2005 University of Maryland Medical Center study found that laughter appeared to increase blood flow by dilating the inner lining of blood vessels, similar to what happens when we exercise. It also brings down levels of the stress hormone cortisol, which has been linked to higher amounts of plaque in carotid arteries and to impairment of learning and memory. The effect of humor on older adults is particularly helpful as an elixir for whole-person wellness for all these reasons.

Laughter improved the release of natural killer (NK) cell activity in a study of cancer patients. Because laughter lowers stress hormones and increases immune cells, the body enjoys sound health, and fewer colds and illnesses, in the short and long term. Laughter also releases endorphins, the body's natural "feel-good" chemicals. This effect can be particularly useful to caregivers who suffer from pain due to stress, whether it is headaches or other chronic ailments. The increased oxygen flow, that relaxes muscles when we laugh, provides us with a shock absorber to get through the long journey of mental, emotional, and physical exertion required to care for the Alzheimer's patient.

Laughter adds more joy and excitement to life, eases anger and fear, improves mood, and enhances resilience. Resilience is especially needed when caretaking extends beyond a year or two. Social health is an important aspect of mental health, and humor strengthens this area by improving relationships, attracting others to us, helping to diffuse conflict, and promoting teamwork. These benefits are especially important for maintaining a bond with one's loved one, and for creating a network of friends to support us.

Humor helps us see our life from a new perspective, and it can enable us to come up with creative solutions to our problems. It raises our consciousness and energy level and can serve to enhance our spiritual connection amidst times of turmoil. If we can remember that change is life's way of sustaining itself, maybe we can supplement the daily grind of caregiving with the amazing human asset called laughter.

Ways to integrate humor into your life

People's sense of humor differs and only you can be the judge of what you find funny, so become aware of what makes you smile, chuckle, and have deep belly laughs. Take note of them so you can do them more often. In the meantime, below are some ideas to get you started.

Movies, Video Clips, and Comedians

Watch cute or funny videos for a mood boost. Watching funny babies and funny animal clips are always a guarantee for a good laugh. You can find hundreds of clips of some of the best comedians: The Marx Brothers, Laurel and Hardy, Jerry Seinfeld, Steve Martin, Bob Hope, Woody Allen, and Robin Williams, to name a few. Comedians like Paula Poundstone, who make light of some of their own personal challenges, can be especially beneficial for those who are suffering. You can use an Internet search to find the top funniest movies of all time to rent, even if you've already seen them. Notice and seize any other opportunities for comedic relief. Some local radio stations air a comedy segment every day. Television sitcoms are another option.

Laugh Buddies

One of the best ways to make sure you get a steady dose of laughter is to have a laugh buddy. Even if it's someone you chat with on the phone, find someone you laugh with regularly and capitalize on it. For some it's an old childhood friend, for others a co-worker, and for some it's a family member. Mine is my mother. Sometimes we take for granted the fact that we laugh with this person in general conversations about life and its idiosyncrasies. You are blessed if you can count on a good laugh during most of your conversations with a particular person.

Begin to recognize the giggles this person brings out in you. (It also helps them to feel good when they make you laugh!) Though laughter is often spontaneous, call this person regularly when you need to keep things real. You don't need to roll on the floor in hysterics for these shares to be meaningful. Even when you exchange chuckles, you elevate your mood and cut the edge off of life's seriousness. Notice what kinds of things you laugh about together. Sharing something silly about yourself with a trusted friend can bring loads of laughter to your day and get you out of narrow-minded thinking. Help others laugh at themselves by pointing out an absurdity that they would find humorous. Again, having someone you know and trust is the key. My mother's and my favorite laugh topic is human relationships (particularly of the romantic persuasion). When you take note of the specific people and topics that make you laugh, you begin to form your laughter capital, which you can call on when needed.

It's likely that not all of your relationships have a humorous element, but as you form new ones and deepen current ones, seek humor. One of the reasons my mother makes me laugh so hard is that she's seen a lot when it comes to people and has experienced many of the struggles that I face for the first time. So, when I call her with my latest drama, she helps me to turn my frown upside down by saying it like it is and pointing to the common and often hilarious aspects of my not-so-unique situation.

Self-Generated Laughter

In addition to noticing how others make you laugh, find ways to crack yourself up. I am no comedian, but ever since I was a child, I have loved doing impersonations of people. Aside from my close confidants, these impressions have been mostly in the privacy of my own company. Doing exaggerated versions of quirks I find in others (or in myself) may seem insane to some, but it's actually the makings of sanity. If something that someone does really bothers me, I would much rather laugh about it than cry about it.

Play detective and see what makes you laugh. Maybe it's just thinking about something funny. Improvisation and the use of your whole body are especially useful in blowing off steam. Doing exaggerated imitations of someone or a situation, whether in front of friends or by yourself, can make light of a situation and bring the absurdity into a comical light. Stand in front of a mirror and make weird and ridiculous faces. You will have no choice but to laugh at yourself!

Write a song or poem about the comedic side of your tragedy. This simple exercise will bring forth your creativity and help you feel in control of your situation. I once made up a rap song about a terrible tragedy I faced, using background music I found, and recording it into a digital recorder. The fun is in the doing, even more than in the end result.

I attended a training seminar years ago by a social worker from the District Attorney's office who worked on homicide cases; one of the most emotionally taxing jobs out there. She gave some great tips on how to stay sane while witnessing some of the most gruesome and faith-testing cases imaginable. Keeping a clown nose in her purse reminded her not to take life or herself too seriously, and when she found herself doing so, she would put on the nose, whether in her car, at the grocery store, or at home, to cut the edge. She also enjoyed reading gossip magazines in the bathtub to get lost in the drama of people she didn't know or care about. Those two brilliant ideas are ones I've used myself and have recommended to clients.

Children

Playing with children any chance you get will add lightness and laughter to your day. Kids are so present and they find humor in the simplest things. You can make a funny face at them and they will crack up and make one back at you. When you get out of your head and really get down and play with them, you will find yourself in the awe and lightness of the world.

Laughter will not only help you through your challenges, but it can also bring you closer to your loved one. Try it for yourself and watch it work its magic. Take the chance for some hearty laughs whenever the opportunity presents itself. When your right brain is accessed in this way, you will feel expansive and in touch with yourself and with life.

* * *

Heather Hans *is a visionary, healer, teacher, and author of the book,* The Heart of Self-Love: How to Radiate with Confidence. *Heather is a Licensed Clinical Social Worker and Psychotherapist, Certified Professional Intuitive Coach, Certified Law of Attraction Advanced Practitioner, and holds a certificate in holistic health. She is a member of the National Speakers Association and the National Association of Social Workers, and she has twenty years of experience in holistic healing and goal achievement. She holds Master's Degrees in Social Work and in*

Business Administration. Subscribe to her free weekly videos at <u>heatherhans.com</u>.

* * *

References

Bains, Gurinder Singh, Lee S. Berk, Noha Daher, Everett Lohman, Ernie Schwab, Jerrold Petrofsky, and Pooja Deshpande. 2014. "The effect of humor on short-term memory in older adults: a new component for whole-person wellness." *Advances Journal*. 28(2): 16-24.

Bennett, Mary P., Judith McCann, Lisa Rosenberg, and Janice M. Zellar. 2003. "The effect of mirthful laughter on stress and natural killer cell activity." *Alternative Therapies in Health and Medicine*. 9(2): 38-45.

Fry, William F. and Michael Miller. 2009. "The effect of mirthful laughter on the human cardiovascular system." *Medical Hypotheses*. 73: 636-39.

27

Journaling

𝒫utting pen to paper is a wonderful way to express your fears, joys, worries, and realizations. You can carry a journal with you and not have to wait for your best friend to return your phone call when you feel as though you might explode with frustration and stress. Learn about the benefits—physical, mental, and emotional—and how to get started. Included are fifty writing prompts to inspire you.

"Writing is a form of therapy.
Sometimes I wonder how all those who do not write, compose or paint can manage to escape the madness, the melancholia, the panic fear that is inherent in the human situation."
– Graham Green, *Ways of Escape*

Journal writing is a great way to release stress. Studies have shown that it actually helps increase the level of disease-fighting lymphocytes circulating in the bloodstream. Keeping a personal journal or diary to pour out your frustration, anger, fear, and heartache is a valuable tool for caregivers. It is especially helpful when your therapist or best friend isn't available to listen to you rant about how you "can't take it any more" or how you cried yourself to sleep.

Journaling allows you to express your deepest emotions. It often reveals a surprising discovery of where you've come from and who you have become as a result of caregiving. It enables you to get in touch with your inner wisdom, which can have a profound effect on how you relate to yourself and the person you are caring for.

Journaling reduces stress

You don't have to be a novelist or professional writer to be healed by words. No one has to ever read your words. But the medical community is discovering that writing can have a profound effect on the body, mind, and spirit, especially after experiencing trauma and stress.

James W. Pennebaker, PhD, professor of psychology at the University of Texas in Austin, gives people an assignment to write down their deepest feelings for fifteen or twenty minutes a day for four consecutive days. The results range from a strengthening of the immune systems to transforming one's life.

Researchers at M.D. Anderson Cancer Center, in Houston, found that twenty-one cancer patients slept longer and with fewer interruptions during the night after venting their feelings on paper, compared with twenty-one patients who wrote about their diet and exercise.

A study published in the journal *Nursing Administration Quarterly* found that expressive writing is recognized as having many therapeutic benefits, including fewer stress-related visits to the doctor, improved immune system functioning, reduced blood pressure, fewer days in the hospital, feelings of greater psychological well-being, reduced depression, improved memory and sleep, and faster healing after surgery. When journaling is combined with social networking, there are even more positive results.

Journaling also helps extended family members of sick patients. One study found that family members of critically ill patients who wrote in diaries for three months had lower levels of symptoms related to posttraumatic stress disorder than the control group, and made a faster psychological recovery.

How to start

- Choose writing materials that work for you. There are countless journals and spiral notebooks available, which come in various styles. Choosing the right pen is even more important. It must fit comfortably in your hand and glide effortlessly on the page. Some people enjoy using a felt tip pen, some like the pressure that an old-fashioned fountain pen offers.

- Find a place where you won't be distracted and light a candle, if appropriate. Set an alarm clock or the alarm on your smart phone. Pour out your thoughts for twenty minutes without stopping or worrying about spelling or grammar.

50 writing prompts to get you going

1. I had a strong reaction to . . .
2. In my family we never talked about . . .
3. Last night I dreamed . . .
4. I find joy . . .
5. I feel most secure when . . .
6. In order to take care of myself emotionally . . .
7. I couldn't possibly live without . . .
8. When I met my partner I . . .
9. The thing I miss most . . .
10. The beautiful thing about me is . . .
11. The first time I felt the emotion of guilt . . .
12. I feel guilty . . .
13. My pulse quickened when . . .
14. A time when I did not feel in control was when . . .
15. My spiritual life intensified when . . .
16. I broke the rules when . . .
17. The hallway was silent . . .
18. I wanted so much to . . .
19. When I awake, my first thoughts are . . .
20. Humor helped me get through . . .
21. It was so difficult when I had to let go of . . .
22. Tell me, honey. . .
23. My favorite lie to tell is . . .
24. The most awesome place I've watched the sunrise is . . .
25. Love is . . .
26. My favorite sound is . . .
27. When I look at the stars . . .
28. What is a mistake people often make about me?
29. On my way to work (or gym) this morning . . .
30. My (our) last doctor's appointment . . .
31. I wish I didn't have to . . .

32. The first time I . . .
33. When I dance (sing, play the piano, etc) . . .
34. What three words describe me right now?
35. The last time I cried . . .
36. If I die tomorrow, I want people to remember that I . . .
37. My friends and family were shocked when . . .
38. I realized I was totally wrong about . . .
39. I wish I hadn't lost touch with . . .
40. I'll always remember . . .
41. It's so hard to . . .
42. I never thought . . .
43. I get a lot of pleasure from . . .
44. When I walk in nature . . .
45. I listened to the birds singing this morning . . .
46. When I meditate . . .
47. I pray that . . .
48. My greatest fear is that . . .
49. I wonder what will happen when . . .
50. I don't understand why . . .

Journal Entry July 20, 2003

How many tears can a human being produce?

By **Barbra Cohn**

I don't know why I didn't cry last night. Usually, after a noticeable lapse in Morris's ability to know what to do when performing a simple task — such as making a bagel, lox, and cream cheese sandwich or locating the silverware in the correct drawer instead of searching in the refrigerator — the emotions of pity, compassion, sympathy, disbelief, and shock meld into a tidal wave that rises from my chest, evaporating into a black cloud that shields me from the natural joy of this life on earth. Light turns into black despair, and then I cry.

But I didn't cry last night when Morris came home shaken and terrified because he had walked out of a meeting in the pouring rain, not knowing where he parked his car. He should have exited the building, turned right, and walked straight up the hill to the parking lot. Instead, he took a wrong turn and found himself at the Boulderado Hotel, cold and miserable. Then, I assume, he went back to the meeting where he enlisted a friend to help him.

This is a typical incident for someone with Alzheimer's disease. Apparently, Morris has gotten lost before; at least he indicated so last night. But this is the first time he arrived home frightened. I have to be more vigilant about his outings, making sure we both have our cell phones turned on, and hoping that he remembers how to use it. It's becoming apparent that he won't be able to drive much longer.

So, why didn't I cry last night? After going through the near-death of Oliver, my beloved Scottish terrier; after grieving over the departure of a dear friend; after being depressed and exhausted for a month over the chaos created by a major flood (the second in two years) in the basement of our house, I feel numb. My heart feels no pain because it is immune to pain. I live a life of continuous grieving. I'm immersed in it. I feel like Job, expecting bad things to happen because I understand the future that I must face; which I wish was already filed in my past history folder. I wish I could rip those pages from my memoir and skip over them, as if I were flipping through the pages of a laborious novel.

I didn't' cry last night. After all, how many things can you cry over in one lifetime? Is there a limit to how many tears your body can produce?

I have to admit that I regret not keeping up on my journal while Morris was sick. Since I'm a professional writer, it was too hard to write during the day and then pour my feelings onto a page at night. But I wish that I had the documentation of what we went through, how far we journeyed, and how I changed.

I've been leading a writing group for the past several years, and I'm continually amazed by the self-awareness, the insights, the observations, and the happiness and angst that appear after only twenty minutes of putting pen to paper or, in the case of most of the women, after vigorously tapping the keyboard. We've cried, we've laughed, and we've created a "secret society" in which our words extend no further than the four walls of the room in which we write.

You don't need a writing forum in order to write your deepest memories, gripes, pains, sorrows, hopes, and desires. You can whine away in the space of your car, bedroom, or neighborhood park. The great advantage to pouring your heart out on a writing apparatus, be it a hardcover journal, iPad or laptop, is that it's always ready when you are. You don't have to make an appointment with your best friend or therapist.

* * *

References

Atkinson, Ronda, Tania Hare, Miranda Merriman, and Anne Vogel. 2009. "Therapeutic benefits of expressive writing in an electronic format." *Nursing Administration Quarterly*. 33(3): 212-15.

Backman, Carl Gosta, Richard David Griffiths, and Christina Jones. 2012. "Intensive care diaries and relatives' symptoms of posttraumatic stress disorder after critical illness: a pilot study." *American Journal of Critical Care*. 21(3):172-6.

Baikie, Karen A. and Kay Wilhelm. 2005. "Emotional and physical health benefits of expressive writing." *Advances in Psychiatric Treatment*. 11(5): 338-46.

De Moor, Carl, Janet Sterner, Martica Hall, Carla, Warneke, Amato Zunera, and Lorenzo Cohen. 2002. "A pilot study of the effects of expressive writing on psychological and behavioral adjustment in patients enrolled in a Phase II trial of vaccine therapy for metastatic renal cell carcinoma." *Health Psychology*. 21(6): 615-19.

Pennebaker, James W. *Opening Up: The Healing Power of Expressing Emotions*. (New York, NY: The Guildford Press, 1990).

Wapner, Jessica. 2008. "Blogging: It's Good for You." *Scientific American*. www.scientificamerican.com/article/the-healthy-type.

28

Light and Color Therapy

$\mathcal{D}$*id you ever wake up in the morning and feel attracted to a certain color? Different colors have a unique effect on us and can help us feel better on all levels: physically, emotionally, and psychologically. Here you will find the benefits of light and color therapy, as well as directions for making a light box with color gels to use for yourself and/or your care partner.*

"Colors, like features, follow the changes of the emotions."
– Pablo Picasso

By **Rufina James**

When you are worn and spent from weeks, months, or possibly years of caring for an ailing loved one, it may seem like there is nothing that can rejuvenate the body and refresh the mind other than six months of solid sleep! Wouldn't it be wonderful if there were some way to deeply rejuvenate in just an hour or so, and to soothe aches or pains and restore balance and equilibrium naturally without leaving the house?

There is a way, and it involves something that most of us take for granted. Our world is full of it. All life depends on it, yet most of us don't understand its potency or how much we crave it: light and color.

Light and color together are a fundamental source of life and energy on earth. They are essential to our lives and well-being. If plants or animals are deprived of light, they cease to grow and develop. If humans are deprived of sunlight, we can develop depression and other imbalances, including a vitamin D deficiency.

Although sunlight appears clear to us, it is really made of all colors. When a beam of sunlight splits by passing through a prism, each element gives off characteristic color waves, which are seen as colors. These colors have effects. Colors on the red side of the spectrum are generally stimulating, while colors on the blue side are sedating. Colors are made up of wavelengths. Each color or shade has a slightly unique wavelength. Just as sound waves create pitches and can be tuned to produce unison or harmony, color waves can also be tuned and can tune the body.

Perhaps because the body consists of more space than matter in a pulsating quantum field, it is very responsive to color waves. The body absorbs color through the eyes, and the skin and the aura take it in deeply if applied properly. If any part of the body is weak, the right color in the right place can restore balance. This is the basis of Spectro-Chrome color therapy, also known as *Dinshah Color Therapy*.

The benefits of light and color therapy

Color therapy is used regularly in modern medicine. Blue light is used to treat neonatal jaundice and acne, and has also been shown to be effective in the treatment of rheumatoid arthritis. Bright white full-spectrum light is used to treat some cancers, SAD (seasonal affective disorder), anorexia, bulimia nervosa, insomnia, jetlag, shift working, alcohol and drug dependency, and to reduce overall levels of medication.

A new technique called photodynamic therapy (PDT) has been developed over the past two decades to identify and treat cancer cells with red light. Athletes now use red light to assist them with short, quick bursts of energy, and blue light for a steadier energy output. Pink light has a tranquilizing and calming effect and is widely used in prison holding cells to reduce violent, aggressive, and anxious behavior among prisoners. It seems to work within minutes of exposure. But there is so much more that can be done with color therapy.

Spectro-Chrome color therapy uses the entire visible spectrum of the colors of electromagnetic radiation to restore balance to the human body. It has been used for several centuries quite successfully for many health conditions, and has the potential for affecting almost all health conditions at any age. Color therapy can be used for physical issues, as well as for mental and emotional issues, and over-all relaxation and rejuvenation. Taking care of others can create a situation of unrelenting stress, especially in a home situation where the caregiver can't get away. However, caregivers can brighten up their day, get a bit of relaxation or a short respite, by utilizing color therapy.

Color therapy is being studied for complementary psychiatric treatment. A recent study, "Chromotherapy in the regulation of neurohormonal balance in human brain--complementary application in modern psychiatric treatment" states, "There is evidence that the visible electromagnetic spectrum of light we see as colors can have an impact on human health. The complex process of neurohormonal regulation of circadian rhythms in humans is essential for synchronized interaction and coordination of internal body functions with the environment. Given these facts, it is clear that any shift in circadian rhythm results in neurohormonal imbalance, which consequently could lead to various psychiatric disorders affecting humans. The main hypothesis of chromotherapy is that specific colors of the visible spectrum are activators or inhibitors of complex physiological, biological, and biochemical processes in the human brain, such as the synthesis of various neurohormones." Even in long-standing chronic cases where the condition is advanced and seemingly immutable, color therapy can provide comfort and relief from pain.

How does it work?

It's actually very simple. All colors evolve from light, and light is necessary for life to exist on earth in the forms of solids, liquids, and gases. Research has shown that humans require light as much as plants do. Why? Because we are vibrating, pulsating, energetic beings that respond to the pulsating energy of light waves. Light affects both the physical and etheric bodies. Light travels in waves, similar to sound waves and the waves of the ocean (although light waves oscillate much faster at hundreds of trillions per second).

Sunlight (white light) contains all the colors of the spectrum. All the colors are needed in balanced proportions for optimal health. We generally do not see these colors when we look through sunlight, but given the right conditions, of a rainbow for instance, they become visible. When a beam of light passes through a prism (which could be a rainbow), it is split into seven visible colors by a process called 'refraction'. Essentially, the light waves change speed when they go through the prism (a different medium), producing the color spectrum and becoming visible.

As large as a rainbow may be, the visible color spectrum is actually a narrow band in the cosmic electromagnetic energy spectrum composed of reds, greens, blues, and their combined derivatives. Most colors fall between the ultraviolet and the infrared ranges of energy or vibrations.

Each color has its own particular wavelength and frequency, and generates electrical impulses and magnetic currents (or fields of energy). Each frequency (i.e., color) has certain effects or "attributes" that are usually generated when used on a body (if it is the appropriate color). The electrical impulses and magnetic currents of the colors are prime activators of the biochemical and hormonal processes in the human body. Colors can have either a stimulating or sedating effect, whichever is required to balance the entire system and its organs.

In a 1972 study, John Nash Ott determined that "different lights affect different enzymatic reactions for healing purposes." Science is just beginning to uncover the nature of the quantum energy inside the atom. All atoms, cells, and organs exist as energy, and each has a distinct vibratory frequency, which translates to its own distinct color.

For every organ, as well as atom or cell, there is an energetic level at which the organ functions best. Any significant change from that vibratory rate results in decreased function or pathology. Restoring the appropriate energy level and energy pattern to the body restores the atoms, cells, organs, and chakras back into balance, allowing the body to heal itself.

Although the colors can penetrate cells to some extent, it is the aura that is initially affected by the light. Color therapy affects the aura by reinforcing weak auric areas and calming down excessive activity, essentially balancing it. The aura is able to transmute and transmit the energy inherent in the light waves to the cells — which are generating the aura — effectively carrying energy into the cells.

In Spectro-Chrome color therapy the normal amount of time

needed for a color therapy session is one hour and it is called a "tonation."

How different colors balance various physical, emotional, and psychological complaints

The colors used in Spectro-Chrome are the three primary colors and the three secondary colors along with the six tertiary colors, comprising the twelve colors of the spectrum (standardized by Dinshah according to his Chromatic Scale):

The Three Primary Colors: Red, Green, and Violet

The Three Secondary Colors: Yellow, Blue, and Magenta

The Six Tertiary Colors: Orange, Lemon, Turquoise, Indigo, Purple, and Scarlet

The colors are divided into the two sides of the color spectrum: the INFRA-GREEN and the ULTRA-GREEN, green being the center color. Green is the physical equilibrating color and most courses of color therapy start with green.

Five in-between colors are also available, (red-orange, lemon-green, turquoise-blue, orange-yellow, green-turquoise) and can be created with the filters.

Red, orange, yellow, and lemon occur on the left side of the spectrum before green, and are the INFRA-GREEN colors. Turquoise, blue, indigo, and violet are found on the right side of the spectrum, and are the ULTRA-GREEN colors.

Opposites: As mentioned earlier, each color has specific effects attributed to it. When a color has reverse attributes to another color, it is called its "opposite." These are the colors that are on opposite ends of the spectrum:

Color:	Opposite:
Red	Blue
Orange	Indigo
Yellow	Violet
Lemon	Turquoise
Purple	Scarlet

This is useful to know in working with the colors because if an area is stimulated by one color, it would tend to be calmed by its opposite, i.e. if an area is stimulated by red, it would be calmed by blue.

Green and magenta do not have opposite colors because they are dual aspects of the same frequency. Lemon and turquoise are each made up of green (a full half) making them very similar in effect. However, lemon is used in chronic cases, while turquoise is used for acute conditions.

Spectro-Chrome color therapy functions something like an electrical transformer by shifting and redirecting the electrical impulses that pass through the body:

- The violet end of the spectrum relieves energy overloads.
- The red end stimulates the non-functioning or under-functioning parts of the system.
- The green center provides a stabilizing or neutralizing effect.

Generally speaking, green, the physical equilibrator, or one of its derivatives (turquoise or blue), is used in cold or flu-like disorders — green when there is no fever, turquoise or blue if there is fever. Yellow is used for chronic, persistent disorders. In disorders involving the heart, blood circulation, or reproductive system, purple, magenta, or scarlet are called for.

When one is stressed, has insomnia, or a pressure headache from tension and emotional stress, violet and purple can help calm the pulse. Sometimes green is the color needed to balance and refresh the body. Green is a wonderful equilibrator and does wonders when applied on the front and/or the back of the head.

I have found green to be an incredible rejuvenator. When I was teaching at-risk, hyperactive, and behavior-challenged students in elementary school and dealing with my own fibromyalgia, Chronic Fatigue, and IBS, there were many days when, after work, I didn't have the strength to get out of the car and walk into the house. The distance between the driveway and the door seemed vast, and the slight incline seemed like a mountain!

Ordinary rest did not revive me. What did was tonating under green light for about an hour. I'd feel a shift half way through the tonation. A wave of relaxation came over me and my strength started to return. After that, I could get up and proceed with the rest of the day.

Caregivers often feel drained and spent. Most caregivers rate their stress level as high, and feel they have little to no time left for relaxing with family and friends. When a caregiver needs to provide continuous care for a prolonged period of time without relief, the caregiver is at risk of exhaustion, health problems, and total burnout, very often bringing on a slew of health problems. That's why it is critical that, as a caregiver, you must first take care of yourself.

As hard as it is to find time to relax, it is vital to your mental, emotional, and physical health to find ways to take a break and recharge your batteries. Even a short respite can help. Color therapy could be one of the ways to take a "mini-break." Although a full tonation lasts an hour, even a short session can refresh you. If you can't leave the premises, think of some creative ways to take a "mini color rejuvenation break." If you don't have time for a full tonation, do as much as you can. Could you sneak in a half-hour tonation sometime during the day? Even fifteen minutes on the head and neck can help to calm, soothe, and relax you and your care partner.

Traditionally, color therapy is done with no distractions such as radio, television, or computer screens. Yet, I have found that working on my computer while shining a color on my face and/or body works just as well as when I lie down in a quiet room. Having a television on would be too much of a distraction, but quietly working on a computer or listening to soothing music is no deterrent.

It's even possible to find a color that can soothe both patient and caregiver at the same time. Think of a dining room infused with the tranquility of pink or violet light; a bath with the water reflecting calming indigo tones or balancing, re-charging green; or the relaxing, sleep-inducing rays of purple before bedtime. Creating the right color environment can make life a little easier and more pleasant for both you and your care partner.

How do I choose the right color?

It is important to choose the right color at the right time. Darius Dinshah's comprehensive manual "Let There Be Light – A Practical Manual For Spectro-Chrome Therapy" lists six-hundred conditions, color schedules, charts, and more, and is an invaluable reference guide: www.dinshahhealth.org.

For more information about how to use colors visit: www.DinshahColorTherapy.com.

How to make a light box

Color gels or "filters" from theatrical lighting are used to create the color filters. Originally, colored glass was used, but glass is impractical and difficult to calibrate. Darius Dinshah did a lot of research with Roscolene filters and found excellent correlations to glass. The Roscolene plastic filters are lightweight, easy to use, and economical. Although many new color gels have entered the market, because Dinshah's research is difficult to reproduce, Roscolene filters are still used today.

Making a light box is not difficult or expensive. A durable light box can be constructed of cardboard and a simple aluminum clamp lamp from a hardware store. You might even be lucky enough to find a long, narrow box that an aluminum clamp lamp fits into nicely, and the job is half done.

Detailed instructions are available online:

www.dinshahcolortherapy.com/how-to/how-to-make-a-lightbox-for-color-therapy.

Purchasing color filters

Roscolene filters can be purchased by the sheet (20" x 24") and cut into any size, or you can purchase pre-cut sets in a variety of sizes. Most places that sell filters also sell at least one model of light fixture. For purchasing information visit: www.dinshahcolortherapy.com.

* * *

Rufina James, *MM, is a natural health publisher and holistic health coach. She is editor of* "The Real Essentials Health News" *and has first-hand experience with many chronic conditions and their most effective natural solutions. She can be reached via* www.dinshahcolortherapy.com/contact.

* * *

References

Kovac, Marina, Drazen Kovacevic, Tija Zarkovic Palijan, and Sanja Radeljak. 2008. "Chromotherapy in the regulation of neurohormonal balance in human brain--complementary application in modern psychiatric treatment." *Collegium Antropologicum*. 32(2): 185-8.

Ott, John N. *Health and Light: The Effects of Natural and Artificial Light on Man and Other Living Things*. (CT: Ariel Press, 1972).

29

Meditation

Meditation has been scientifically shown to reduce stress and increase happiness. Here you will learn about the benefits, how you can learn from a certified meditation teacher, and a simple meditation technique to instantly calm yourself down.

"If a person's basic state of mind is serene and calm, then it is possible for this inner peace to overwhelm a painful physical experience." – The Dalai Lama

Morris and I were both teachers and practitioners of Transcendental Meditation™ (TM), as taught by Maharishi Mahesh Yogi. Hundreds of studies have shown that TM helps normalize blood pressure and reduce stress and anxiety. This chapter includes an interview with Dr. David Orme-Johnson, one of the principal researchers in the world on meditation and its effects. Orme-Johnson has published more than one hundred scientific studies in peer-reviewed journals and has reviewed the meditation research on chronic pain and insomnia by a National Institute of Health Technology Assessment conference. He has traveled to more than fifty-six countries to speak about meditation to government officials, members of Congress, heads of state, the press, and others. He is a former consultant for the Center for Natural Medicine and Prevention, which was funded by the NIH-National Center for Complementary and Alternative Medicine.

This chapter also includes insights of a caregiver who found a sense of tranquility through meditation while caring for her mother.

What is Transcendental Meditation?

Transcendental Meditation (TM) as taught by Maharishi Mahesh Yogi is a simple mental technique that is practiced twenty minutes twice a day, morning and evening. It isn't a belief system, and you don't have to sit up straight without a back support. If you can think a thought, you can meditate. Maharishi Mahesh Yogi began his first global tour in 1959, and brought TM to the United States. He achieved fame as the guru to the Beatles, and eventually trained more than forty-thousand TM teachers who taught TM to more than five million people in one hundred and fifty countries. He is considered responsible for the popularization of meditation in the West.

What are the benefits of TM?

The main reason that people practice TM is for stress relief. After learning how to meditate, practitioners typically worry less, have less tension and more energy, and are able to deal with stressful situations more calmly. Once the sharp edge of stress is removed, meditators enjoy restful sleep, a more positive outlook, and are able to think more clearly. More than three hundred and fifty research studies have verified that the daily practice of the TM technique produces a wide range of positive effects on a person's mind, body, and behavior.

Interview with Dr. David Orme-Johnson

Q: What happens during Transcendental Meditation?

During the twenty minute meditation, practitioners experience transcendental consciousness, commonly called "restful alertness." Physiologists refer to this as a wakeful hypo-metabolic state, characterized by decreased metabolic activity and increased EEG (brain wave) coherence. The body experiences a deep state of relaxation because activity in the sympathetic nervous system is reduced. The blood vessels are dilated and heart rate is lowered. There is a reduction in stress hormones, including adrenaline, noradrenaline, and cortisol.

Breathing slows down, not due to a drop in metabolic rate, as was previously thought, but because of a significant drop in the respiratory exchange ratio (the ratio of the amount of carbon dioxide produced by the body to the amount of oxygen consumed). The breath slows down by as much as forty percent, and is sometimes suspended for up to a minute, without any need to gasp afterwards in order to take in extra air. It is interesting to note that this reduced responsiveness to carbon dioxide levels during deep meditation may be an indication of increased equanimity, said to be a quality that develops with regular practice of the Transcendental Meditation program.

One of the changes in the brain that appears to be correlated with increased bliss during transcendental consciousness is increased EEG coherence. During periods of marked slowing of the breath and transcendental consciousness, EEG coherence increases across all frequencies and cortical areas of the brain compared to periods immediately before and after. Such patterns do not occur in people who are just resting and deliberately holding their breath.

The evidence indicates that the state of increased EEG coherence seen during the Transcendental Meditation program becomes a trait of increased coherence outside of meditation and during tasks. Other studies found that resting EEG coherence increased after two weeks of TM practice, and that during a reaction time test, the participants had higher EEG coherence when compared to individuals who did not meditate.

Dr. Keith Wallace was the first person to measure the physiology of transcendental consciousness. He found that its physiological pattern validates it as a fourth major state of consciousness, which is physiologically distinct from the first three major states: waking, dreaming, and sleeping.

Q: What is the benefit for caregivers?

People who meditate are able to cope more easily with stress. A study at the University of California at Irvine showed that Transcendental Meditation reduces the brain's reaction to stress. In this pilot study, twelve subjects practicing TM for thirty years showed a forty to fifty percent lower brain response to stress and pain compared to twelve healthy controls. Further, when the controls then learned and practiced Transcendental Meditation for five months, their brain responses to stress and pain also decreased by a comparable forty to fifty percent. This study shows that you don't need to practice TM for years and years until you experience benefits. Even after meditating for a brief length of time, meditators report that they feel more energetic and relaxed, and experience deeper, more restful sleep than before.Additionally, high blood pressure, which is directly correlated to stress, has been shown to be significantly reduced in patients who practice TM.

A meta-analysis (examination of numerous studies) of six hundred TM research papers found that, overall, TM is more effective than most typical and alternative treatments for patients with high anxiety, including chronic anxiety and post-traumatic stress disorder.

My personal experience, and the experiences of many meditators that I've taught and know, is that whether or not one experiences transcendental consciousness during the Transcendental Meditation program depends upon the condition of the physiology. Transcendental consciousness is a state of perfect balance. If the physiology is out of balance due to fatigue, eating too much, eating too little, too much or too little of anything, chronic or acute diseases, or long-term stresses, then meditation works on normalizing these imbalances.

Q: Is the Transcendental Meditation Program a Religion?

Millions of people have learned the Transcendental Meditation program from all religious faiths, including priests, rabbis, and ministers, and they find no conflict between the practice and their religion. Instead, they find that the Transcendental Meditation program enriches the practice of their own religion. In addition, many teachers of the Transcendental Meditation program are ordained clergy in traditional religions and, at the same time, continue to teach the technique.

It should be pointed out that the Federal Government has never declared that the TM program is a religion. In fact, over the last twenty-five years, numerous government programs involving the TM program have been approved by the Federal and State governments, implementing or researching the TM program in health facilities, schools, universities, research facilities, prisons, and probation programs. More than approximately twenty million dollars in government grants have been provided for these purposes.

Q: How can you learn to meditate?

Visit this site to locate a teacher near you and to learn about the seven steps to learning the practice. www.tm.org/learn-tm.

Notes from a caregiver who practiced TM (4/6/2012)

Mummy and I had been alone since my dad died when I was seven years old. It was sudden and shocking.

When I graduated from college, I started Transcendental Meditation and my mom started TM about three months after I did. It was a lifesaver for both of us. She said she did not have her anxiety attacks anymore, her health issues cleared up, and she felt happier.

Mummy came to live with my husband Phil and me when our first child was about a year old. That was thirty-eight years ago. She was my friend, my nanny, my helper, my confidant, and my mum. It was "mother at home" all the time, every day. She worked at her jobs, she helped with the house, and she was my only girlfriend. She sewed, fixed, listened, saved, loved, and honored our privacy.

Fast forward to 2003 when Mummy's health started to fail. And then the dementia started, and I began to lose my best friend. The best times were when we could do our TM meditation together and I knew that was keeping both of us strong and in touch. I know that without TM we would not have made it through that tough time when she began to slip away and was aware of the slipping. Just sitting and meditating together really helped us to know that even though she was declining, we were healing in the process.

Now she does not remember who she really is and who I am. I have been angry and still go through the anger, the sadness, the frustration, and guilt. All this growth is taking time, love, and help from my Phil and my boys, my family, friends, counselors, and even strangers. Thankfully, I still have TM. I have time for myself when I can go deep into my own bliss, into my Self, and experience that part of us that can never change and I can know that Mum is there too. It is very comforting.

A quick meditation for instant relief

Although this five to ten minute sitting meditation will not provide the profound physiological changes or stress reduction provided by practicing Transcendental Meditation, it might help take the edge off a disturbing event and emotional response.

1. First, scan your body for how your muscles feel. Start at your head and move downward. Move your head gently from side to side and try to relax your neck muscles. Move your shoulders up and down and drop them instead of keeping them hunched. Make circles with your shoulders, one at a time, and then together. Roll them forward and backwards. Pretend you are turning a doorknob open and closed with your hands. Move from your neck down to your torso. Feel any sensations of heat in your chest, and go further down, releasing tension in your belly and pelvis. Open and close your thighs, and then flex and release your feet by crunching your toes and releasing them. Allow yourself to feel all the body sensations. Are your muscles heavy and warm? Warm your hands together if they are cold.

2. Focus on your thoughts. Are they scattered, worried, up-setting? Feel the emotion associated with them. Do you feel sad, hurt, angry, fearful?

3. Try to replace those disturbing thoughts with ones that are comforting. Picture yourself on a warm, sunny beach where you can hear the waves hitting the shore. Or, think of a time you and a loved one had a picnic in a lovely meadow and the afternoon was beautiful and carefree. Hold that pleasant thought for a moment.

4. How do you feel now? Content? Peaceful? Happy?

5. Fill your body with that happy emotion and let it filter through your muscles like a beam of light. Take three complete breaths, in and out. Breathe in and out, and on the last exhale let the light radiate outward through your nostrils. Now carry that beam of happy sunshine into your activity and let it surround those you interact with the rest of the day.

* * *

References

Anderson, James W., Carolyn Gaylord-King, Sanford I. Nidich, Maxwell V. Rainforth, John W. Salerno, and Roberto H. Schneider. 2007. "Stress reduction programs in patients with elevated blood pressure: a systematic review and meta-analysis." *Current Hypertension Reports.* 9(6): 520-8.

Arenander, Alarik, Joe Tecce, Fred Travis, and R. Keith Wallace. 2002. "Patterns of EEG coherence, power, and contingent negative variation characterize the integration of transcendental and waking states." *Biological Psychology.* 61(3): 293-319.

Badawi, Kheireddine, Robert Keith Wallace, David Orme-Johnson, and Anne Marie Rouzere. 1984. "Electrophysiologic characteristics of respiratory suspension periods occurring during the practice of the Transcendental Meditation program." *Psychosomatic Medicine.* 46(3): 267-76.

Barnes, VA and David Orme-Johnson. 2012. "Prevention and Treatment of Cardiovascular Disease in Adolescents and Adults through the Transcendental Meditation® Program: A Research Review Update." *Current Hypertension Reports.* 8(3): 227-42.

Barnes, VA and David Orme-Johnson. 2014. "Effects of the transcendental meditation technique on trait anxiety: a meta-analysis of randomized controlled trials." *Journal of Alternative and Complementary Medicine.* 20(5): 330-41.

Benson, Herbert, Robert Keith Wallace, and Archie F. Wilson. 1971. "A wakeful hypometabolic physiologic state." *American Journal of Psychology.* 221(3): 795-99.

Bronson, Edward C., and Michael C. Dillbeck. 1981. "Short-term longitudinal effects of the Transcendental Meditation technique on EEG power and coherence." *International Journal of Neuroscience.* 14(3-4): 147-51.

Farrow, John T. and Russell J. Herbert. 1982. "Breath suspension during the Transcendental Meditation technique." *Psychosomatic Medicine.* 44(1): 133-53.

Frederick, Travis and Keith R. Wallace. 1999. "Autonomic and EEG patterns during eyes-closed rest and Transcendental Meditation (TM) practice: A basis for a neural model of TM practice." *Consciousness and Cognition.* 8(3): 302-18.

Haynes, Christopher T. and David W. Orme-Johnson. 1981."EEG phase coherence, pure consciousness, creativity and TM-Sidhi experiences." *International Journal of Neuroscience.* 13(4):211-7.

Orme-Johnson, David. 1977. "EEG coherence during transcendental consciousness." *Electroencephalography and Clinical Neurophysiology.* 43(4):E 487.

Orme-Johnson, David. 2006. "Neuroimaging Laboratory, University of California at Irvine."*NeuroReport.*

Severeide CJ. "Physiological and phenomenological aspects of Transcendental Meditation." In: Chalmers RA, Clements G, Schenkluhn H, Weinless M, editors. *Scientific Research on Maharishi's Transcendental Meditation and TM-Sidhi Program*: Collected papers. Vlodrop, the Netherlands: Maharishi Vedic University Press, 1979/1989.

Travis, Frederick and Robert Keith Wallace. 1997. "Autonomic patterns during respiration suspensions: Possible markers of Transcendental Consciousness." *Psychophysiology* 34(1): 39-46.

Wallace, Robert Keith. 1970. "Physiological effects of Transcendental Meditation." *Science*. 167(3926): 1751-1754.

Wallace, Robert Keith. 1972. "The Physiology of Meditation." *Scientific American*. 226(2): 84-90.

30

Music Therapy

Music is the universal language, stress diffuser, up-lifter, bonder, and natural medicine. Music can evoke memories, increase social interaction in people with dementia, and help them form trust with their caregivers. Learn also how different tempos can affect the body and mood.

"Music… can name the unnameable
and communicate the unknowable." – Leonard Bernstein

The Power of Music

By **Michelle Pelc**

Anyone who knew Morris was keenly aware of his passion for music. Throughout his two years at Juniper Village, Morris could often be found strutting around with his headphones on. Many times when I would arrive for a visit I could hear him singing in his room from down the hall.

The summer before he passed, I took him to the Boulder Creek Festival, an annual event that encompasses food, rides, music, and a plethora of vendors. I thought Morris would love the live music, but I was a bit apprehensive that it might be too crowded and over stimulating for him. When we arrived my suspicions were realized; it was so packed with people that it was difficult to walk. We made our way through the crowd and I held Morris's arm, verbally guiding him down the path. It was flooded with people walking in all directions, and he seemed anxious as he held my arm tightly and struggled to find the words to express his dismay. I considered just turning around and taking him to a nearby ice cream shop.

We took a few more steps, nearing the stage where a band started to play. The music was loud and I decided it was too much and we needed to leave. Just as I was about to tell this to Morris he stopped and said, "I think I, I'm going to have to...going to have to..." I was ready for him to say get out of here when instead his shoulders started bouncing to the beat of the music. He let go of my arm, and danced into the crowd. Once he got going he couldn't stop. I was in awe of how freely he moved; shaking his hips, turning in circles, waving his hands, arms, legs, and shrugging his shoulders. He danced exuding pure joy!

* * *

Michelle Pelc, MA, earned her Masters degree in Transpersonal Counseling Psychology from Naropa University in 2010. She has eight plus years of professional and personal experience working in long-term care, adhering to a holistic approach while attending to the emotional, mental, and physical well-being of her clients. Currently, she serves as a Case Manager for seniors both in their homes and care facilities specializing in Alzheimer's and Dementia Care privately and with Windhorse Elder Care. Michelle can be reached at michellem.pelc@gmail.com.

* * *

It's true that Morris loved music. He went through dozens of batteries for his CD player, and at least a half dozen CD players and headphones in the last several years of his life. The music made him happy, and the feeling was contagious. As Morris walked through Juniper Village the staff would often stop to listen and sing along. Eventually, staff would play Morris's CDs in the dining room where he ate so everyone could enjoy the music.

Music helped Morris maintain his dignity and uplift his spirit, especially when nothing else seemed to work. I am especially grateful to music therapist Laurie Rugenstein who played guitar and sang for Morris at the end of his life. Her lovely voice and playing soothed him and me during a difficult time.

Music Therapy

Rebekah Stewart, MA, MT-BC
Neurologic Music Therapist

"What exactly *is* music therapy?" This is quite a familiar question to board-certified music therapists like myself. The power of music is not generally a concept that most individuals need to be convinced of; however understanding *why* music can work so well as a therapeutic tool is often where more explanation and education is needed. This chapter will explore a brief scientific explanation behind the use of music therapy with dementia populations, the ways music can help caregivers both connect with, and provide higher quality of life for, their care partners and how music can be used as a personal self-care tool.

For centuries, people have been fascinated by the power of music and its unique and prominent role in cultures and societies worldwide. This fascination has grown into a unique field of study known as Music Neuroscience. Music neuroscientists' sole focus is how music affects the human brain and behavior, and a major area of study focuses on music, memory, and dementia. The general public's fascination with this has also grown recently due to the appearance of films and internet videos which show elderly individuals "coming alive" again when favorite music from their past is played for them.

Why does this happen? We now know that people's ability to retain and recall memories related to music is preserved much longer than many other skills during the progression of Alzheimer's disease. Simply put, the main reasons for this are twofold:

1. Memories connected to music often contain a stronger emotional component,which helps the brain to more effectively store and then recall the information.

2. Recent studies show that when people listen to preferred music, the music brings back memories that are often connected with a strong, generally positive emotion. People remember music that they like. Usually that music is tied to autobiographical memories such as the song that was played for the first dance at their wedding.

The areas in the brain responsible for musical memory processing and recall are not affected as early into the disease as other areas of the brain. Additionally, so many parts of our brains are involved in processing music that during memory tasks involving music, healthier areas of the brain can assist areas with more damage.

There is some additional research that suggests that goal-oriented music therapy groups can temporarily improve an individual's cognitive function, and decrease anxiety and negative behaviors often associated with dementia. Also, caregiver singing and inter-action during difficult self-care tasks (dressing, bathing, hygiene, meals) significantly decreased the patient's anxiety and negative behaviors and increased positive social interaction between the caregiver and care partner.

When I worked at a skilled nursing facility specializing in late stage dementia care, I had the great privilege of meeting a couple named Bruce and Katy *(names have been changed for patient privacy). Katy was no longer able to communicate effectively; her words and sentences were mostly nonsensical. However, when Bruce and Katy came to my music therapy group, Katy knew all the words to the songs and she and Bruce could sing together. She was often able to utter an intelligible sentence following the close of the song as well, such as "thank you dear," or "that was nice." In that moment the music was able to facilitate a human connection, sometimes between Bruce and Katy, sometimes between Katy and myself. In her younger years, Katy had been a proficient pianist. When she sat down to play, even in the months leading up to her death, she could still play *Clair de Lune* and Beethoven (her favorite composer) better than I ever will.

Music engagement can help you connect with your loved ones and care partner. Oxytocin, the chemical in our brain that is re-leased during intimate interactions such as breastfeeding and in-tercourse, helps us to form trust and bonds with other humans. It is fascinating that this chemical is also emitted when people sing and make music together. This truly should come as no surprise. When you engage in music making with your care partner, wheth-er it's dancing, singing, playing, etc., it can create an incredible meaningful bonding experience. When caregivers participated in a music therapy group with their care partners, caregivers re-ported increased satisfaction with visits and interactions, and the researchers noted an increase in positive social behaviors on the part of the care partners as well.

Dancing to music that carries special significance can be a wonderful way to interact with your care partner. There was this young couple, Peter and Sally,* and although Peter could no longer speak and generally spent his days wandering the hallway, when Sally visited him, she would sing and they would dance together down the hallway. Peter's face always lit up when they were dancing. In the same way, Mimi and Teddi*, a mother and daughter, would dance during the weekly swing band concert held at the facility where Mimi lived. Teddi never missed those concerts because it was one of the most positive hours of interaction she got to have with her mother every week.

In addition to dancing, active music making (singing, instrument play, songwriting) is another wonderful way to interact with your care partner. Ted,* a client of mine, suffered from younger onset Alzheimer's disease. He and his wife Hillary* were the parents of two young children, so in addition to dealing with the life changes that went with the diagnosis, they were also in the midst of parenting. Ted thoroughly enjoyed drumming during our sessions and I suggested that he and his family attend a drum circle as a way to interact and spend time with one another. This became an activity that they continued to do, and a wonderful way for Ted to spend time with his children and simply be "Dad."

Active music making can be another way to not only create space for meaningful interaction, but can also be a highly effective stress reliever for caregivers and/or their care partners. Active music making can relieve tension, boost immune responses, and decrease cortisol, the body's stress hormone. Our bodies produce cortisol in response to stress, and too much cortisol can disrupt our immune system, making it more likely that we will get sick or fatigued.

As a caregiver, practicing self-care is one of the most important things you can do for yourself. Using music to interact with your loved one can be a fantastic way to relieve stress; however sometimes it is useful to engage in some practices alone. As stated above, active music making decreases cortisol levels in our bodies, and if this is something that is comfortable for you, it can be extremely effective. Spend time writing songs, playing your

instrument, or singing. However, there are more passive ways
of using music as a self-care tool, and one of the most common is
relaxation. As with all relaxation practices, it is important to create
a space where you are free from distraction, and allow yourself
enough time to be fully present. It is also important to select the
right music, which is different for every individual. What is relaxing for one may not necessarily be relaxing for another.

1. **Slower consistent tempo**
   The average human resting heart rate is somewhere between sixty to one hundred beats per minute (bpm). Our
   physiologic responses entrain to tempo in music, which
   means that our respiratory and heart rates naturally speed
   up or slow down to match the tempo of the music we listen to. Relaxing music should have a speed that matches
   a resting heart rate and it should remain relatively consistent.

2. **Softer dynamics**
   Most people can agree that extremely loud music is more
   jarring than softer music (although this is not the case for
   every individual- these characteristics are just general
   guidelines).

3. **Very little dynamic variation**
   Going from loud to soft and soft to loud is not conducive
   to relaxation. It is unexpected and often very startling;
   enough to raise your heart rate just when you were about
   to fall asleep! Dynamic levels should be consistent so
   there are no unexpected surprises to snap you out of your
   desired state.

4. **Predictable harmonic structure**
   Most of us have been surrounded by culturally western
   music paradigms since birth. Our brains have been trained
   to expect music to progress and end in certain predictable
   ways (this is called the "Theory of Expectations"). If you
   listen to some 20th century modern classical music, you
   will immediately see what I am talking about; none of it
   sounds "right." This lack of predictable and expected patterns keeps your brain guessing, and when your brain is

trying to constantly figure out what's going on, it is completely counterproductive to being able to relax.

Music has a wonderful way of helping us connect with people, access significant memories, improve our mood, and decrease stress. Even in the midst of caring for a loved one suffering from a degenerative disease such as Alzheimer's, music can be used in many different ways as a tool to improve the quality of life for both caregivers and care partners.

*   *   *

Rebekah Stewart, MA, MT-BC is a board certified Music Therapist and Neurologic Music Therapist. Rebekah has experience working with interdisciplinary treatment teams, and initiated the first ongoing interdisciplinary collaborations between the music therapy and rehabilitation departments at Garden Terrace at Overland Park, Kansas – an Alzheimer's Center of Excellence. Rebekah maintains an active membership in the American Music Therapy Association and currently serves as the Continuing Education Committee Representative for the Midwestern Region. She can be reached at: Rebekah@rrmusictherapy.com.

*   *   *

References

Bittman, B., Berk, L., Felten, D., Westengard, J., Simonton, O., Pappas, J., & Ninehousder, M. (2001). Composite effects of group drumming music therapy on modulation of neuroendocrine-immune parameters in normal subjects. *Journal of Alternative Therapy*, 38-47.

Brotons, M. & Pickett-Cooper, P. (1996). The effects of music therapy intervention on agitation behaviors of Alzheimer's disease patients. *Journal of Music Therapy, 33(1)*, 2-18.

Bruer, R., Spitznagel, E. & Cloninger, C. (2007). The temporal limits of cognitive change from music therapy in elderly persons with dementia or dementia-like cognitive impairment: A randomized controlled trial. *Journal of Music Therapy, 44(4)*, 308-328.

Ceccato, E., Vigato, G., Bonetto, C., Bevilacqua, A., Pizziolo, P., Crociani, S., Zanfretta, E., Pollini, L., Caneva, P., Baldin, L., Frongillo, C., Signorini, A., Demoro, S. & Barchi, E. (2012). STAM protocol in Dementia: A multicenter, single-blind, randomized, and controlled trial. *American Journal of Alzheimer's Disease and Other Dementias, 27(5)*, 301-310.

Clair, A. & Ebberts, A. (1997). The effects of music therapy on interactions between family caregivers and their care receivers with late stage dementia. *Journal of Music Therapy, 34(3)* 148-164.

Garcia, J., Iodice, R., Carro, J., Sanchez, J., Palmero, F. & Mateos, A. (2011). Improvement of autobiographic memory recovery by means of sad music in Alzheimer's disease type dementia. *Aging Clinical and Experimental Research, 24(3),* 227-232.

Guetin, S., Fortet, F., Picot, M.C., Pommie, C., Messaudi, M., Djabelkir, L., Olsen, L.L., Cano, M.M., Lecourt, E. & Touchon, J. (2009). Effect of music therapy on anxiety and depression in patients with Alzheimer's type dementia: Randomised, controlled study. *Dementia and Geriatric Cognitive Disorders, 28,* 36-46.

Haj, M., Postal, V. & Allain, P. (2012). Music enhances autobiographical memory in mild Alzheimer's disease. *Educational Gerontology, 38,* 30-41.

Hammar, L., Emami, A., Gotell, E. & Engstrom, G. (2011). The impact of caregivers' singing on expressions of emotion and resistance during morning care situations in persons with dementia: An intervention in dementia care. *Journal of Clinical Nursing, 20,* 969-978

Koyama, M., Wachi, M., Utsuyama, M., Bittman, B., Hirokawa, K., & Kitagawa, M. (2009). Recreational music-making modulates immunological responses and mood states in older adults. *Journal of Medical and Dental Sciences, 56(2),* 57-70.

Levetin, D. J. (1997). *This is your brain on music: The science of a human obsession.* London, UK: Penguin/Sage Publishing.

Simmons-Stern, N., Budson, A. & Ally, B. (2010). Music as a memory enhancer in patients with Alzheimer's disease. *Neuropsychologia, 48(10),* 3164-3167.

Stalinski, S. & Schellenberg, E. (2012). Listeners remember music they like. *Journal of Experimental Psychology: Learning, Memory, and Cognition.* 1-17.

Tan, X., Yowler, C., Super, D. and Fratianne, R. (2012). The interplay of preference, familiarity, and psychophysical properties in defining relaxation music. *Journal of Music Therapy, 49(2),* 150-179.

Van de Winckel, A., Feys, H., Weerdt, W. & Dom, R. (2004). Cognitive and behavioral effects of music-based exercises in patients with dementia. *Clinical Rehabilitation, 18,* 253-260.

31

Nutritional Support for Caregivers

Food is medicine. It can heal us, and it can also harm us if we don't choose the right foods. Dr. Ed Bauman provides the guidelines for creating a diet of holistic, chemical-free foods so you can stay healthy and strong. Included are nutritious and delicious recipes, and herbs that produce a calming effect.

"Let food be thy medicine and medicine be thy food"
– Hippocrates

Dr. Ed Bauman is the author of the Eating 4 Health™ model, which emphasizes eating:

- Whole, fresh, and unrefined foods
- Organic, chemical-free foods
- A variety of foods (think colors of the rainbow)
- Seasonal foods, including produce that is in season
- Pure beverages, including filtered water and herbal teas, fresh vegetable and fruit juices, mineral broths
- Booster foods such as seaweed, nutritional yeast, spices, seeds, nuts, and algae
- SOUL foods—Seasonal, Organic, Unadulterated (Unprocessed), and Local

Seasonal Eating

- Winter: Increase your protein and fat intake
- Spring: Increase intake of whole grains and greens
- Summer: Eat more fruits and salads
- Fall: Emphasize more whole grains and root vegetables (carrots, beets, squash)

Prevent Burnout with Delicious, Healthy Foods and Stress-reducing Habits

By **Edward Bauman**, EdM, PhD

Caregivers are predisposed to helping others and not caring for themselves. It starts with the morning routine. If you're a caregiver, how much time do you have to do something nurturing for yourself? Prayer, meditation, exercise, and preparing your own food for the day are a great way to start. Most people get up, get a cup of coffee, and have cereal or a muffin and run out of the house or immediately begin their caregiving duties. Or, they get their coffee and muffin or doughnut on the run.

Start the day with a great breakfast

The alternative is to make some hot cereal (quinoa, oatmeal, buckwheat, 7-grain), and add nuts and seeds for protein and quality fats, and dried or fresh fruit such as berries. Then you can add spices, such as cinnamon, nutmeg, and ginger, for added flavor and nutrition, and a one-half to one teaspoon serving of honey, molasses, or maple syrup instead of sugar or an artificial sweetener. Maybe you add a nutritional powder, a balanced blend of digestible proteins, fats, carbohydrates, vitamins, minerals, trace elements, natural enzymes, and friendly flora that provides the energy you need for optimal performance without caffeine or stimulants. You can also have some yogurt, cottage cheese, or kefir, which would build a more nutrient-rich breakfast.

Eggs make a delicious, fast breakfast, and they are terrific for the brain — particularly the yolk — regardless of cholesterol issues. Buy hormone-free, free-range eggs if possible, and when you cook them, keep the yolk on the soft side. The yolk has fatty acids that help protect the brain, as well as B vitamins and choline. These vitamins support acetylcholine, which helps to support memory. Have greens with the eggs, in an omelet or as a side. Spinach, kale, Swiss chard, etc. provide fiber, chlorophyll, vitamins, and minerals. Or you can add a mix of yellow and red peppers, and shitake mushrooms and onions for a nourishing, protective breakfast that provides healthy fats, fiber, and protein.

If you like, toast corn tortillas or a gluten-free bread made from sprouted grains. Or you can have brown rice or another grain, such as quinoa, millet, buckwheat, or barley with eggs and a green veggie. Then you have a delicious morning meal that will feed your hormones and their neurotransmitters, and support healthy blood sugar for three to four hours so you can show up for a care partner and stay stable because you didn't have caffeine and carbs for breakfast.

If you have a weak digestive system, you can take a digestive enzyme. Or you could try different teas: black, green, white, red, or herbal. Tea has less caffeine and more antioxidants and minerals than coffee. The minerals and the bioflavonoids in tea are protective against the environmental stress of caregiving, and help support the nervous system, which is going to be challenged in a high-demand situation. Tea is an important beverage for recovery and rejuvenation. Green tea, especially, is excellent. It is slightly caffeinated and supplies numerous antioxidants. So any type of tea is better than coffee.

The important thing is to stay hydrated. Have non-caffeinated, unsweetened beverages throughout the day, particularly water and tea. The rule of thumb is to have 48 to 64 ounces of non-sweetened, non-artificially sweetened drinks. Hydration keeps the body in proper pH (how acidic or alkaline your body is) and protects it from getting dehydrated, which is a cause of inflammation and other kinds of imbalances.

Meal planning

Caregivers need a plan for what they're going to eat when caring for people. A well-nourished person can deal with higher levels of crisis and decision-making, and stay in relationship during troubling times. Undernourished people don't function as well. Their stress load becomes more burdensome on their organs, and their reserves of nutrients become depleted.

What happens when caregivers aren't able to prepare their own meals?

They need help. If the caregiver has low energy or is depressed, they need another person in their support system, such as a nutrition consultant or a natural chef who can make food for them or get food for them from a natural foods deli, or teach them to eat differently rather than relying on comfort food.

Dangers of the Standard American Diet (SAD)

It's not called SAD for nothing. It's higher in calories, lower in nutrients, and depends on sugar, stimulants, and pick-me-up foods. It also feeds exhaustion and depression. Taking vitamins might help, but supplements aren't sufficient if the diet and lifestyle are unhealthy.

Caregivers might need to create a schedule where they get more time off so they can rest and have time to handle the food for themselves and their care partner. It's worth every penny to have professionals come in to help with the person who has Alzheimer's, so the caregiver can get several hours during the day when she or he is not on the job, because the emotional involvement of caregiving is exhausting.

Caregivers need to have other activities and health practices. Dance, practice yoga, take a cooking class, or participate in a spiritual group activity that is not focused on caregiving, but is focused on self renewal. Co-dependence is typical in a caregiving situation, in which you spend more of your energy on someone else to the detriment of caring for yourself. In some situations, caregivers don't eat enough. It might be helpful to eat snacks every few hours, including quality proteins, fats, minerals, vitamins, and antioxidants.

Healthy snacks

Here are some ideas for a healthy snack: hummus, guacamole, or a yogurt and spinach dip with raw veggies (carrots, celery, cucumbers, red peppers) are all things that are easy to make at home, even if you're busy. Almonds, cashews, walnuts, and filberts are good to have on hand. Two to four ounces of nuts, preferably raw or dry roasted, are great as a snack or added to a veggie dish for increased protein content.

Caregivers can make smoothies for breakfast or snacks, or occasionally as a quick meal if they can't sit down to enjoy one. Use a protein powder made with whey or hemp; a fiber such as flax or chia seeds; dried coconut for texture and taste; fresh or dried fruit, such as banana or berries or dates; and herbs and spices such as fresh ginger, turmeric powder or turmeric root, or cinnamon to taste. Blend all this together with organic milk, a nut milk, coconut milk, or fresh fruit juice. You can also add avocado for its creamy texture and healthy fat. Make a large pitcher of smoothie mix (2-4 cups), which you can have morning and afternoon, or after a long day. In warm weather, you can put a smoothie mixture in popsicle molds or ice cube trays for a finger dessert.

Any of these foods can be given to patients. In some cases, people will eat a lot, and in other cases these types of food are new and different and need to be introduced slowly and gradually.

Nutritional soups

Soup makes an inexpensive meal and can be made, stored, and enjoyed for several days. A homemade soup is far more nourishing than canned soups, which are overcooked, high in sodium, and can have additives and preservatives. A lentil or split pea soup, or chicken soup with veggies, is easy to make and can be eaten any time of day. The addition of sea vegetables (wakame, hiziki, arame, kombu) provides a good source of minerals and natural salts, and supports endocrine function, particularly the thyroid.

Nutritional yeast is another excellent booster food, which is high in B vitamins, chromium, and selenium. This yellow, flaky powder can be sprinkled like Parmesan cheese on soup, toast, brown rice, or any food. It adds flavor and is very energizing for people who are tired and depressed.

How does food affect your mood?

Neurotransmitters are the brain chemicals that communicate information throughout your brain and body. The brain uses neurotransmitters to tell your heart to beat, your lungs to breathe, and your stomach to digest. They can also affect mood, sleep, concentration, and weight, and can cause adverse symptoms when they are out of balance. Neurotransmitter levels can be depleted many ways. It is estimated that eighty-six percent of Americans have suboptimal neurotransmitter levels. Stress, poor diet, protein deficiency, poor digestion, poor blood sugar control, drugs (prescription and recreational), alcohol, and caffeine can deplete them.

Serotonin is necessary for a stable mood. A deficiency can result in depression, insomnia, binge eating, and carbohydrate craving. Activities that enhance serotonin involve cross crawl movement, as in swimming, hiking, and biking.

Dopamine keeps us focused and motivated. Dopamine is sometimes referred to as a "gas pedal" neurotransmitter. Activities like listening to rock & roll music, tennis, rock climbing, action sports, and attending an exciting show or concert enhance these neurotransmitters. Too much can result in aggressive behavior. When in balance, dopamine increases alertness, wakefulness, and energy. Deep breathing, weight bearing exercise, and strength training all enhance dopamine. Sugar, cigarettes, and other addictions deplete dopamine. Norepinephrine is responsible for stimulatory responses in the body. Dopamine converts into norepinephrine and they are considered a single chemical.

GABA keeps us feeling "balanced." Too many carbs and refined foods deplete GABA. Exercise, being outdoors, and paying attention to your personal needs are important. Passion flower, lemon balm, and valerian help support GABA, and help you fall asleep if your mind is on over-drive.

How to boost your neurotransmitters

- Eat a serving of high-quality protein with every meal and snack.
- Focus on complex carbohydrates and eliminate junk foods (refined carbs).
- Enjoy unlimited amounts of fresh veggies.
- Eat a good breakfast!
- Eat three balanced meals and one or two snacks/day.

Natural mood boosters

At night, having a lighter dinner after eating three or four meals and snacks during the day will improve sleep and enable you to wake in the morning with a good appetite. Usually people get wired and tired when they eat lightly during the day, have a big dinner, and then snack at night. The outcome is they don't sleep well and aren't hungry in the morning. This can lead to depression, exhaustion, fatigue, and poor stress management.

Having soup and salad and a grain that is high in magnesium and B vitamins at night can help improve insomnia. In some cases, nutritional supplementation in the day with meals and at night before bed, with the help of a professional nutrition counselor, is advisable.

For depression, EFAs (essential fatty acids) are particularly important. Most people will need a supplement with two to three grams of omega fatty acids per day. Other nutrients to consider are vitamin D3, which calms the nerves and supports calcium metabolism, or a multi-vitamin, if someone has had a lifetime of poor nutrition.

Vitamin B complex is important for stress reduction. Foods that provide B vitamins and magnesium include: whole grains, nutritional yeast, fresh fruits, dark leafy greens, and protein-rich foods.

Beverages

People ask how much liquid do I need each day? Of course, that will vary due to activity levels, age, health status, and the water balance in the foods a person eats. One who eats more fresh fruits and vegetables will need less fluid than one who eats meats, cheese, and breads. In general, I suggest four ounces of fluid each hour, sipped slowly to allow for a slow and steady hydration of the body.

My recipe for stress management and withdrawal from addictive substances is to have a cup of herbal tea when a craving comes along. Take time out to boil the water, steep the tea, and enjoy the natural flavor and aroma of the herbs, while writing in a journal what is bothering you. This is a good way to process and nourish yourself rather than reaching for something less healthy.

Ruby Chai*

Wake up to this stimulating yet non-caffeinated version of chai (serves 2)

(*From *Flavors of Health Cookbook* by Edward Bauman, EdM, PhD & Lizette Marx. Bauman College Press, 2012.)

Ingredients

- 1 cup filtered water
- 8 green cardamom pods
- 6 whole black peppercorns
- 1 ¼-inch slices fresh ginger, peeled and diced
- 1 2-inch stick cinnamon
- 2 whole cloves
- 1 star anise pod
- 2 cups almond milk or coconut milk
- 1 tablespoon maple syrup
- 2 tablespoons rooibos (red tea) or 2 rooibos tea bags

Method

1. Put water and spices in a saucepan and bring to a boil. Reduce the heat to low and simmer for 20 minutes.

2. Add milk and maple syrup and heat to a strong simmer. Do not allow to boil.

3. Add the tea and turn off the heat. Allow to steep for 5 minutes, then strain chai into heatproof mugs.

Almond Milk (1 serving)

Blend or shake well together:

- 1/3 cup almonds (ground)
- 2 Tbsp. honey
- 1 cup purified water or grain milks (soy, rice, and oat)
- Dash almond or vanilla extract
- Variations:
- Add raisins or dates to taste

Can substitute almonds with any nuts or seeds.

Add various spices to taste, such as cinnamon, coriander, ginger, cardamom or basil.

Herbs produce a calming effect

Herbs or adaptogens can be helpful for increasing energy without stimulation. An adaptogen is a natural substance — usually an herb — that helps the body adapt to stress by producing a calming effect on the whole physiology. Phytosterols, the plant compounds in the herbs ashwaghanda, gotu kola, passion flower, schizandra, skullcap, rhodiola, and cordyceps have been scientifically shown to support the adrenal glands and healthy blood chemistry, and enhance the body's ability to resist the ravages of stress. Valerian, Siberian ginseng, kava kava, oat straw, and hops also help reduce stress.

As we age, the adrenal glands and endocrine system can become deficient. This neuro-hormonal depletion is a result of chronic stress and inadequate nutrition, and most caregivers are running on empty. By becoming more grounded and stable, caregivers could have an easier time caring for themselves while caring for others.

Herbal teas to prevent stress*

(*from *Recipes & Remedies For Rejuvenation Cookbook* by Edward Bauman, EdM, PhD, Bauman College, 2005)

Emotional Stabilizer (4 servings)

A drink for overwrought and stressed-out folks

Add 2 Tbsp of each herb per liter of water for some or a combination of all of the following herbs. Steep in boiled water 20-30 minutes:

- Oat straw
- Kelp
- Elecampane
- Comfrey
- Rosemary

- Eucalyptus leaves
- Licorice or star Anise
- Mint

Do not use licorice if you have high blood pressure!

These herbs can be found at a natural foods store or online at a bulk herb and spice shop.

Trace Elements Tea (4 servings)

Very soothing to the nervous system and an overstressed body.

Add 2 Tbsp of each herb per liter of water for some or a combination of all of the following herbs. Steep in boiled water 20-30 minutes:

- Alfalfa
- Fennel
- Seaweed
- Nettle watercress
- Slippery elm

Mineral Broth (8 servings)

This broth helps alkalinize the body and warm the system. It also helps counter the negative effects of stress. Have it as a bowl of soup, or sip it throughout the day.

Wash with a scrub brush and cut into 1-inch chunks:

- 2 cups yams
- 1 medium potato (any variety, raw with skin)
- 1 cup zucchini
- 1 cup cabbage
- 1 cup green beans
- 2 cups celery

Slice into strips:

- 1 cup collard greens
- 1 cup onion

Coarsely chop:

- ½ tsp. fresh parsley

- ½ tsp. dill weed
- 1 clove garlic

Add whole:

- ½ cup flax seed

Place ingredients in a large pot with a lid.

Cover with filtered water, just to the level of the vegetables, and add:

- 6 slices fresh ginger root
- ¼ cup or more seaweed (dulse, nori, wakame, hiziki, kombu)
- Seasonal greens (kale, mustard, spinach, or broccoli)

Bring the water to a boil, then turn down to a simmer, and cover for three to five hours. Strain the broth with a colander. Let cool before refrigerating or freezing. Will keep in fridge for five to seven days or in the freezer for four months.

Variations:

- Add cubed sweet potato to soup mix in the beginning of cooking time.
- Add ½ tsp. curry 10 minutes before serving for a zesty flavor.

Middle Eastern Rejuvenation Dinner (8 servings)

Boost your immune system in the winter with this easy and delicious meal.

Tomato Vegetable Soup

- 2 cans whole tomatoes (organic, chopped)
- 2 onions (sautéed)
- 6 cloves garlic (pressed and sautéed)
- ½ tsp. oregano (dried)
- 1 medium winter squash (peeled and cut into chunks)
- 1 medium rutabaga (chopped)
- 1 bunch turnips (chopped greens and roots)
- 1 pound zucchini (cut into chunks)

Add water to cover and simmer until done. Serve with brown rice or couscous.

Moroccan Lentils with Sweet Potatoes (8 servings)

Great side dish or can be served as a main dish with a fresh salad and bread.

In a heavy stockpot, fill with:

- 5 cups chicken or vegetable stock

Add and simmer 30 minutes:

- 2 cups lentils (dry)
- 2 large cloves garlic (minced)

Then turn off the heat, cover the pot, and let sit for 45 minutes to 1 hour.

Meanwhile, prep the vegetables:

- 2 medium onions (chopped)
- 2 medium carrots (peeled and chopped)
- 3 whole tomatoes (fresh or canned, peeled, and chopped)
- 1 pound sweet potatoes (peeled and cubed)

After the lentils have sat, add the chopped vegetables and the spices:

- 1 Tbsp. cumin seed (roasted and ground, or just use powdered cumin seed)
- ½ tsp. ginger (ground)
- ½ tsp. tamari sauce (low sodium)
- ½ tsp. coarse or sea salt
- ¼ tsp. black pepper (freshly ground)
- cayenne to taste

Cover and cook until the sweet potatoes are tender. Adjust seasonings to suit your taste. Can be served hot or at room temperature. Top with ½ bunch cilantro or Italian parsley (chopped).

* * *

Edward Bauman, EdM, PhD is the Founder and President of Bauman College Holistic Nutrition and Culinary Arts. He is a groundbreaking leader in the field of whole foods nutrition, holistic health, and community health promotion. Dr. Bauman is working to bring the Eating for Health approach to community agencies and clinical health care settings, both locally and nationally. He can be reached via: ed.bauman@baumancollege.org.

32

Self-Massage

Find out how to do a luxurious self-massage in the privacy of your home. Tips for creating a relaxing environment, affirmations for setting the tone, and specific oils are included, as well as how to give a massage to your care partner.

"Within you there is a stillness and a sanctuary to which you can retreat at any time and be yourself." – Hermann Hesse

By **Stephanie McAdams** RN, BSN

One solution to combating stress is to incorporate practical wellness regimens that *feel* nurturing and restorative to the whole person. An aromatic oil self-massage can become a time of refreshing respite from the tasks and demands of caregiving. Regular self-massage is a simple, economical, and practical way for caregivers to enhance their physical, mental, and spiritual health, and to promote self-awareness and improve the mind-body-spirit connection.

Hippocrates, the founding father of Western Medicine, recommended various wellness regimens and said, "A perfumed bath and a scented massage every day is the way to good health." Historical women including Hatsheput, the first female pharaoh of Egypt, Queen Esther of the Old Testament, and Cleopatra, used perfumed oils as part of their daily regimen.

Marguerite Maury, an Austrian born biochemist (1895-1968), is considered the pioneer of modern day aromatherapy. She believed in an individualized, holistic approach to healing, and her research — which was based on aspects of Ayurveda and Traditional Chinese Medicine (TCM) — demonstrated the effects of essential oils on the whole person. Maury recognized the therapeutic value of creating unique, personalized blends of essential oils diluted in vegetable oil carriers to promote one's physical, emotional, mental, and spiritual well-being. She emphasized that the aromatic oil blends should be externally applied by massage.

Abhyanga, which means both oil and love in Sanskrit, has a long and celebrated history in Ayurvedic medicine (see chapter 20, *Ayurveda*). For thousands of years, people in India have used abhyanga oil massage as a way to maintain health, support restful sleep, and increase longevity. It is still prescribed by practitioners today.

Ayurveda's theory is that the physiological effects of the application of oil on the body are similar to the effects produced when one is saturated with "love." Both experiences impart sensations of stability, warmth, and comfort. It is believed that oil massage produces healthy skin, facilitates physical movement of joints and muscles, alleviates joint stiffness, acts as a passive form of exercise by increasing circulation, helps the process of removing waste, and relaxes the body. For the best physical, psychological, and spiritual results, it is recommended that oil massage be performed daily. A quote from Charaka Samhita, an ancient classical Ayurvedic text states:

> "The body of one who uses massage regularly does not become affected much even if subjected to accidental injuries or strenuous work ... By using oil massage daily, a person is endowed with pleasant touch, trimmed body parts, and becomes strong, charming, and least affected by old age."

One of the principle aspects of Ayurvedic massage is to incorporate aromatic oils. The ancient texts tell us that jasmine was used as a general tonic for the entire body. Rose was employed as an antidepressant and used to strengthen the liver. Chamomile was used for headaches, dizziness, and colds. Many of the properties ascribed to herbs and aromatic oils by the ancients are regarded as valid today.

Oil massage neutralizes stress

Skin, the largest sense organ of the body, is the immediate recipient of an oil massage. A quarter size piece of skin contains more than three million cells, twelve feet of nerves, one hundred sweat glands, fifty nerve endings, and three feet of blood vessels. It is estimated that there are approximately fifty receptors per one hundred square centimeters, which totals nine hundred sensory receptors throughout the human body. Our skin is essentially a giant complex communication system that carries messages from the external environment to the internal body, mind, and spirit. It is no wonder that oil massage has profound positive effects such as stimulating circulation of blood and lymph, dispersing nutrients, removing metabolic wastes, reducing pain, and enhancing relaxation.

Massaging warm oil over the skin helps to calm the nervous system, and a calmer nervous system is less likely to trigger the release of stress hormones. This results in numerous positive outcomes, and is so beneficial to caregivers and their care partners.

After receiving a ten minute foot massage each day for two weeks, people with dementia and a history of agitation immediately showed a significant decrease in agitated behavior, according to recent research. In addition, the reduction in agitated behavior remained significant for two weeks after the massage intervention had ended. The study, "Exploring the effect of foot massage on agitated behaviors in older people with dementia: A pilot study," involved twenty-two people with a diagnosis of dementia and a history of clinically significant agitation. The mean age of the subjects in this study was about eighty-five years, and all of them were permanent residents of a care facility.

Massage works just as well for caregivers. A small pilot study of nineteen staff members who provided direct care to residents with dementia indicated that when caregivers received up to three ten minute foot massages per week for four weeks, they experienced improved mood, reduced anxiety, and lower blood pressure.

A study with acute care hospital nurses who received regular massages for five weeks demonstrated that they had lower urinary cortisol levels, lower blood pressure readings, and lower reported stress compared with the control group who did not receive massage.

Other research shows that essential oils blended into massage oil helps reduce stress and anxiety and is beneficial to the immune system. A study done in Thailand examined the effect of a blended oil of lavender and bergamot oils on forty healthy volunteers. The subjects rated themselves as calmer, more relaxed, and less anxious than the control group that did not receive the massage.

Massage oils

Effective massage typically requires a lubricant to reduce friction and supply slippage, and it is best to use pure oils and fats that come from the nuts and seeds of plants notable for their health benefits to the skin. Nuts and seeds contain the energy potential of plants, which explains why many vegetable oils are so nutritious. Several key ingredients make certain plant oils highly beneficial to the body. Among these nutrients are essential fatty acids. Phospholipids, another key ingredient present in vegetable oils, are especially important in nourishing the fatty myelin sheath covering nerve cells. Lecithin contains emulsifiers that help the body break down fats. Sterols are also present in many vegetable oils and have been shown to have anti-inflammatory effects. The phytoestrogens and isoflavones present in many oils have been noted to help reduce the levels of free estrogen in women's bodies, inhibiting breast cancer growth. Lastly, many vegetable oils contain varying degrees of vitamins A, B, C, E, and K.

Which carrier oil should you use?

- Sweet almond oil is light and penetrates easily, making it an excellent aromatherapy carrier oil. It contains essential fatty acids and vitamins, and offers healing properties for dry, inflamed, itchy skin.

- Argan oil comes from the seeds of the Moroccan Argan tree. It is one of the richest sources of vitamin E and contains a large percentage of unsaturated fatty acids and antioxidants. It is said to prevent premature aging of the skin.

- Coconut and olive oils are cooling and are best used in summer. Olive oil helps sooth inflamed skin. Coconut oil is very light, has a pleasant smell, and washes out of linens easily.

- Grape seed oil contains vitamins, minerals, and essential fatty acids. It is light and an excellent carrier for aromatherapy oils.

- Sesame is a heavy warming oil, and is recommended for use in the cooler months.

- Jojoba oil has antioxidant properties and contains myristic acid, a natural anti-inflammatory that helps relieve arthritis symptoms.

Choosing essential oils

The next critical step in creating aromatic therapeutic massage oil is to add essential oils. Carrier oils typically lack a pleasant odor and blending them with essential oils can make the oil massage a truly sensual and mood altering experience. Ultimately, the goal is to create a fragrant aromatic oil that evokes the sensations of pleasure and overall well-being. (Please refer to Chapter 18 - *Aromatherapy* to learn about specific essential oils and their effects.)

Ready-made aromatherapy massage oils are available in natural foods and supplement shops. Or you can make your own.

How to blend the oils

1. Fill a sterile glass jar (opaque or a dark color is best) with the carrier oil of your choice.

2. Use an eyedropper to put fifteen to twenty drops of essential oils in the bottle of carrier oil. Start out with a small number of drops. You can always add more.

3. Gently swirl the oils in the jar. Do not stir or shake. Store oils away from heat or light in an airtight opaque or dark colored glass. Label the oil for future use.

Self-massage

Self-massage is economically practical and an excellent way for caregivers to take an active part in their own healing and stress management. The bonus is that once caregivers learn how to massage themselves, they can apply this skill to massaging their care partner.

Benefits of self-massage

- Many people are uncomfortable with their bodies. By doing regular self-massage, one gains an understanding of his or her body.

- From a holistic nursing perspective, self-massage promotes enhanced self-care, enhanced self-empowerment, enhanced self-awareness, and enhanced body-mind-spirit connection. All of these elements are crucial in the optimization of one's personal development, health, and well-being. Another benefit of self-massage is the spiritual aspect of applying oils to the body, otherwise known as *anointing*. This practice dates back thousands of years, and is by no means limited to a particular culture or religious tradition. There are almost three hundred references to the practice of anointing in the Judeo and Christian Bibles. In the New Testament, oil symbolizes the Holy Spirit and is even referred to as the "oil of gladness" and the "oil of joy."

Ancient Egyptians also practiced the ritual of anointing and believed the effects included promotion, protection, physical healing, restoration of spiritual well-being, and even assistance into the afterlife. Today, people of various faiths and traditions continue to anoint with oils, testifying to its beneficial effects. Self-massage offers a perfect opportunity to enhance one's spirituality by including the recitation of a prayer, blessing or affirmation, or setting a simple intention prior to and throughout the oil massage.

A personal empowering affirmation can either be chanted mentally or verbally throughout the oil massage. One suggestion is simply chanting 'love' which comes directly from part of the Ayurvedic definition of abhyanga, as discussed previously. Here are some other affirmations that are especially appropriate for caregivers:

- I only speak loving words to my care partner.
- I have unbounded energy and patience today.
- I feel strong and healthy.
- My mind is at peace.
- I pay close attention to my body's needs.
- I send love and appreciation to all the cells in my body.
- Healing energy flows through every cell in my body.
- I am thankful for my many blessings.
- I am cheerful and happy.
- I am grateful for my loving friends and family.

How to do the massage

Here are a few basic guidelines. Of course, according to your personal preference or for practical reasons, you can make slight adjustments. Ideally, aromatic oil self-massage should be done in the morning before bathing and exercise. Since our bodies, minds, and spirits benefit from regular routines, try to use the same pattern during most of the massages. For practical reasons, many people prefer doing the aromatic massage after bathing.

But doing it any time during the day will still be beneficial. Plan to do the massage for a minimum of five minutes, up to twenty minutes. The longer the time, the more beneficial the massage will be. No matter when or how long you do it, you will reap benefits.

1. Heat a liberal amount of oil by placing the bottle of oil in a pan of warm to hot water. Avoid using the microwave, if possible.

2. Effleurage (light pressure, soothing strokes) is the type of massage recommended, but slightly more pressure can be applied, depending on personal preference and health status.

3. It is important to stroke the body moving in a distal to proximal direction, which means stroking should be towards the heart. The extremities should be massaged prior to the trunk. Begin with the legs first.

4. Circular massage movement is used over all the joints, and long upward strokes are used over the long bones.

5. It is difficult to massage one's back, but attempt to massage as much of the lower spine as possible, and the backs of the shoulders and upper scapula.

6. Massage the chest and abdomen using gentle, broad, clockwise, circular strokes. When massaging the abdomen, follow the path of the large intestine, moving up on the right side, then across, then down on the left side.

7. If time is limited, at least massage the feet. It is also recommended that the scalp be massaged at least once a week. In this case, for obvious reasons, it may be best to shampoo hair following oil massage. Massaging the feet and scalp with oil is thought to relax the entire body.

8. For women who have not yet incorporated self-breast exams into their routines, this practice of self-massage is an ideal time to begin.

Contraindications

There are times when oil massage is contraindicated. Examples of contraindication are: broken or infected skin, skin rash, swollen or tender areas, masses, active cancer, phlebitis, thrombosis, infection, fevers, or flu. Pregnant women and individuals with health conditions or chronic disease should consult their physicians before incorporating daily aromatic self-oil massage into their health regimen.

A practical tool for slowing down and connecting with your care partner

Practicing regular aromatic oil self-massage helps us to slow down and provides us with a time to nourish our bodies and relax our minds. Daily aromatic oil self-massage promotes self-awareness and enhances the mind-body-spirit connection. Practically speaking, it helps us get to know our bodies and become more comfortable in the skin we live in. It can even be a therapeutic diagnostic where we may notice any unusual changes in our bodies that warrant medical attention. Regular aromatic oil self-massage is a simple, economical, and practical way for caregivers to enhance their own physical, mental, and spiritual health, as well as their care partner's. It provides the opportunity to intimately connect with a care partner on the level of touch.

The Encyclopedia of Essential Oils: The Complete Guide to the Use of Aromatic Oils in Herbalism, Health, and Well-Being by Julia Lawless, June 1, 2013, Conari Press.

* * *

Stephanie H. McAdams *RN, BSN, RYT is a registered nurse and certified integrative aromatherapist who has studied the holistic healing therapies of aromatherapy, yoga, Ayurveda, and energy medicine. One of the primary tools Stephanie shares is aromatic oil self-massage.Contact Stephanie at* yourbodyizatemple@gmail.com.

* * *

References

Ackley, Betty and Gail B Ladwig. *Nursing Diagnosis Handbook, An Evidence-Based Guide to Planning Care (8th ed).* (St. Louis, MO: Mosby Elsevier Inc., 2008).

Bull, Ruah, and Joni Keim Loughran. *Aromatherapy & Anointing Oils, Spiritual Blessings, Ceremonies, and Affirmations.* (Berkley, CA: Frog Books, 2001).

Burne Johnston, Amy Nicole, Wendy Moyle, and Siobhan Therese O'Dwyer. 2011. "Foot Massage Decreases Agitation in Dementia Patients." *Australian Journal on Aging.* 30(3): 159-161.

Cooke, Marie, Amy Johnston, Wendy Moyle, Jenny Murfield, and Billy Sung. 2013. "The effect of foot massage on long-term care staff working with older people with dementia: a pilot, parallel group, randomized controlled trial." *BMC Nursing.* 12(5).

Dossey, Barbara Montgomery and Lynn Keegan. *Holistic Nursing: A Handbook for Practice (5th ed).* (Sudbury, MA: Jones and Bartlett Publishers, LLC, 2009).

Hongratanaworakit, Tapanee. 2011. "Aroma-therapeutic effects of massage blended essential oils on humans." *Natural Product Communications.* 6(8): 1199-204.

Jones, Elizabeth Ann. *Awaken to Healing Fragrance, the Power of Essential Oil Therapy.* (Berkely, CA: North Atlantic Books, 2010).

Kusmirek, Jan. *Liquid Sunshine, Vegetable Oils for Aromatherapy*. (Italy: Floramicus, 2002).

Robbi, ND Zeck. *The Blossoming Heart, Aromatherapy for Healing and Transformation*. (Victoria, Australia: Aroma Tours, 2004).

Svoboda, Robert E. *Lessons & Lectures on Ayurveda*. (Albuquerque, NM: The Ayurvedic Press, 2008).

Welch, Claudia. *Balance Your Hormones, Balance Your Life: Achieving Optimal Health and Wellness through Ayurveda, Chinese Medicine, and Western Science*. (Philadelphia, PA: Perseus Books Group, 2011).

33

Sound Therapy

ound therapy has been used since the beginning of time as a tool for healing. Just the right sound can have a profound healing effect on our physiology. Researchers have demonstrated that sound helps to facilitate shifts in our brainwaves by using entrainment. Entrainment synchronizes our brainwaves by providing a stable frequency that the brainwave can attune to. This results in our brainwaves shifting from a waking state of consciousness to a relaxed state, a meditative state, and/or sleep, where deep healing can take place. Learn how to create sacred sounds with crystal bowls, how to listen for sounds in nature, and about recordings that you and your care partner can listen to together.

"Do you know that our soul is composed of harmony?"
– Leonardo da Vinci, *Notebooks* (1451-1519)

The Healing Transformative Power of Sacred Sounds: Energetic Tools for Families and Caregivers of Alzheimer's Patients

By **Marianne W. Green**

We didn't know each other. She came with a friend. When Barbra walked into my Sacred Sound meditation group the first time, I read deep sorrow in her eyes. In the next ninety minutes, after a long inner journey supported by sacred sounds, there was some sharing and I learned that her beloved husband had Alzheimer's. Barbra appeared to be young — too young to have a husband with Alzheimer's I thought, and I felt compassion in my heart.

Before beginning a Sound meditation, we tune into the intention of the session. An intention is a vibrational signature of purpose and energy, which amplifies the energies of the sound vibrations. My intention with groups is always that I be guided to play the combinations of sounds that will support the highest good of everyone in the room. These sound meditations are 'inspired' spherical improvisations, played on crystal and Tibetan bowls, chimes, koto, Monochord, and other instruments with rich overtones.

Ninety minutes later as Barbra was leaving, her essential self radiated through her eyes when she hugged me. I felt the connection of one soul to another; both recognizing that she had been led back into her own sacred space, into the embrace of the power of universal love. She had reconnected with Source Energy, with Love and Light. Some call this God. Some call it the Power of Infinite Possibilities, and some call it The Creation or All That Is.

Meditation with Sacred Sounds, which I call Spherical Improvisations, is one of atonement with The Creator and brings harmony, transcendence, and deep healing of the Soul.

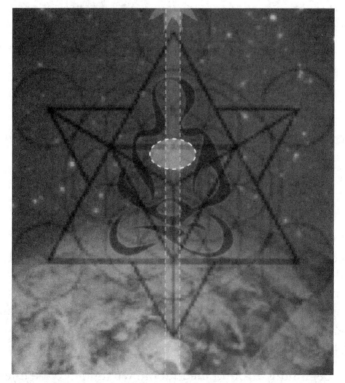

Human Vibrational Field. December, 2015.
Created by Marianne Greene.

Sacred Sounds are quintessential in aligning the vibrational field of humans. This picture exemplifies the alignment of the physical and subtle energy field of humans. This picture also exemplifies the alignment of the physical and subtle energy fields with the vertical energy where heaven and earth unite in the heart, integrating us with our divinity.

Spherical Improvisations – work with the healing sounds
and imagery – is based on the premises
that Sacred Sounds lower our brain waves,
ease us out of the grip of our mind and emotions,
unify our vibrational field and guide us into Presence.
the Vertical Energy: Connection
-with Mother Earth,
-with our Own Innate Nature,
-and with Source Energy: Love and Light

Many paths can gently lead us to this inner connection. Sacred Sounds, also called Healing Sounds, are part of our humanness. Our breath, our voice, sounds of nature, instruments of aboriginal tribes such as drums, rattles, primitive horns (the didgeridoo), the ankh, bells, and chimes, just to name a few, have been used for ages in healing ceremonies.

Seers, ancient yogis, and Chinese doctors have understood that humans are vibrational beings. Special video equipment can even track the colors of the subtle energy field (aura) of a person who is asked highly charged questions that evoke emotional responses, showing how the physical body and the aura are affected. In sound therapy it is the vibration of the instrument, along with the intention, that is quintessential in aligning the vibrational field of humans.

Vibration and Quantum Physics

The following is an introduction to our 'energetic being.' I invite you to read it slowly and out loud, since words and the intention behind them are strong vibrations. Everything is energy!

Quantum Physics is teaching us that everything is a complex organization of sub-atomic, pulsating vibration. Our cells and organs are amazing compositions of frequencies, overtones, harmonics, and resonances: our own personal orchestra.

Scientific studies have proven that certain music and specific sounds and intervals (like a fundamental tone and another tone higher or lower together with that tone) have very stimulating, balancing, or even sedative effects on our physical, emotional, mental, and spiritual bodies.

Sounds with rich overtones – our own voice, special instruments like harps, singing bowls, tuning forks, didgeridoos – align our brain hemispheres, lower our brainwaves and blood pressure, harmonize our cells, and strengthen our immune system. Sounds can be used as a potent form of vibrational acupuncture, dissipating energy blocks so that energy flows freely in our physical body and subtle energy fields.

Sacred Sounds, toning, chanting, and kirtan (group chanting) move us into the field of pure vibration outside of our minds and feelings. Special overtone instruments can lead us swiftly and directly into silence, where we reconnect with our soul and with that state of pure consciousness where we are not bound by emotions or repetitive and imprinted thoughts.

Your Higher Self, the core of your being, communicates with you in the form of vibrational messages. Colorful symbols and visions are the language of light. They are encoded with layers of information and insights that have the ability to release and transform energy, emotion, and thought at a conscious and cellular level.

Sacred Sounds align you to your highest luminous self. They enliven your innate knowledge that you are a co-creative being. This reconnecting to the core of your being is the ultimate healing for you - and ultimately for our world. We reconnect to that field of LOVE AND LIGHT, Source Energy, or 'I AM' Presence, as some would call it. Reconnecting is 'At-ONE-ment with the Creation, with Source Energy.' This is what brings harmony, transcendence, and deep healing of the soul.

Individual sacred sound sessions

Sacred Healing Sound sessions, especially when scheduled regularly, can be extremely beneficial to an individual who is overwhelmed with the sadness, grief, non-acceptance, and exhaustion of all the difficulties that accompany caring for a loved one in any sort of major short or long-term challenge.

Lying on a massage table during a healing sound session is a beautiful and rejuvenating experience. Setting your intention helps to intensify the power of the rich overtones of the Sacred Sounds as they interact with your physical body and subtle energy fields (emotional, mental, and spiritual), dissipating stress and negative, scattered energy.

If you are unable to go to a sound therapist, there are many excellent recordings that you can use for one of these deep realignments. Many men and women love my CD *"Soul's Garden."* Jonathan Goldman's *"Crystal Bowls Chakra Chants"* and *"Waves of Light"* and *"Dreamtime"* by Hemisync are my favorites. Good sound healing recordings are unique in that they have been 'composed' to clear and balance with *intention* and a profound understanding of the energetic and physiological interactions of sounds and overtones.

An interactive session with the client and a sound healer can sometimes result in a lasting transformation of grief into acceptance and solace. I remember a young woman who had recently lost her mother. I heard the grief in her voice on the telephone, as she told me that the previous day she had erased the very last voice mail from her mother that she had been saving. Linda *(name changed)* asked if she could come for a sound session.

Linda arrived and there were tears, but gradually her whole Being began to shift and lighten as the healing sounds soothed the sadness and realigned her to her bright, divine, and eternal SELF. In this particular session, I urged her to ask her Higher Self for a symbolic image of her mother. Accompanied by my healing sounds, colors in hand, she proceeded to draw a beautiful flower in a lovely garden. The picture glowed with love, as did Linda's eyes. She left my studio transformed.

I have met Linda at different times over the years, and she has repeatedly declared that that day was a turning point in her grief process.

Healing sounds help edit emotional and mental "files"

As holographic vibrational beings, we have a dense physical energy body with more subtle fields around us: the emotional, mental, and spiritual bodies. Think of these bodies as digital computer files in our sub-conscious realm, which can be opened and closed and even deleted. I like to describe our *emotional body* as the part of us that energetically remembers all the feelings we have ever experienced. It is like one giant computer folder with files dating back much longer than we can remember. Some of these "files" have been edited and reedited by inner work and energy work. Depending on the extensiveness of our conscious inner explorations, many files have also been deleted.

For instance, there might be a file called *"pain when I think of my mother who, because of Alzheimer's, doesn't know me anymore."* A thought or the feeling that my mother doesn't know me anymore can open this file. So we have a thought and a connected emotion and the release of stress hormones. Pain. A vibration. Our field is now aligned to pain. We could perhaps take a pill that would temporarily close the files that have been opened. They are still there. But we could also take another route: witness our pain, share this openly with a loving companion, go for a walk in nature (and be supported by the amazing healing powers from Mother Earth, Gaia), play some soothing music, breathe slowly, do the HeartMath® Coherence meditation (see page 260), and every so often seek out a therapist. A sound therapist would play the sounds for you that will not close the files, but will help edit them, and perhaps when you are ready, will even delete them. The vibration of the healing sounds is the tool to energetic release and higher consciousness. For instance, the file *"my mother doesn't recognize me anymore,"* opened and ready for the first edit, might go something like this: *"my mother doesn't recognize me anymore and this is so painful for me. I allow myself to feel pain. I am so sad. I observe the pain. Who is observing the pain?"*

Healing sounds can assist one in moving from the space of being controlled by the pain, to the space of becoming the conscious observer of the pain. Energetically something else happens: the healing sounds realign the field (body, emotions, mind, and soul) that has been in deep distress. Slowly, a sense of coherence, calmness, and peace are achieved. Energetically there is a new holographic alignment because that file has now been edited and saved as: *"I, now realigned with my Higher Self, observe my pain when my mother doesn't recognize me."* The body energetically remembers this new alignment. The next time this file is opened, there will be a new neural pathway forming in the brain, with slightly different hormones being released. You are on the healing path to wholeness with a new opportunity to further edit the file.

Coherence

My experience has been that deep slow breathing, combined with very slow, spacious tones (as for instance with singing bowls), stabilizes your heart rate and synchronizes and lowers your brain waves, establishing coherence between heart and brain. The tuning fork exercises, singing DO and SO, listening to *Soul's Garden* or Hemi-Sync® recordings (a trademarked brand name for a process used to create audio patterns that induce brainwave synchronization) are positive tools to ease us out of the incoherence of stressful emotional states. Aligning the heart and brain establishes an even more powerful state of coherence.

I heard someone state so beautifully that when your heart is filled with gratitude and appreciation the emotional body has no hunger, and in my words there is no occasion to reopen these files. The Institute of HeartMath® teaches that when we are feeling appreciation *in our hearts*, and when we direct that appreciation towards something or someone, ourselves included, we initiate coherence between our brain and heart.

Deep slow breathing, combined with very slow, spacious tones (as for instance with singing bowls), stabilizes your heart rate and synchronizes and lowers your brain waves, establishing coherence between heart and brain. You move from polarity and the feeling of separateness into coherence, into the feeling of unity, and into presence, as Eckhart Tolle teaches. This is our essence, our connection with the eternal, with Love and Light.

Many studies have focused on the effect that musical tempi have on our heart rate. My own personal experiences, and those of my students and clients, have left no doubt in my mind that Sacred Sounds support the heart breathing exercises which are the foundation of the coherence between heart and brain. The following appreciation practice anchors coherence.

HeartMath® Appreciation Tool™

(generously supplied by the HeartMath® Institute)

1. **Heart Breathing**

   Focus your attention on your heart area, and breathe a little deeper than normal, in for 5 or 6 seconds and out 5 or 6 seconds.

2. **Heart Focus**

   Imagine breathing through your heart. Picture yourself slowly breathing in and out through your heart area.

3. **Heart Feeling**

   Activate a positive feeling as you maintain your heart focus and breathing. Recall a time you felt good inside, and try to re-experience the feeling. Remember a special place or the love you feel for a close friend, relative or treasured pet. The key is to focus on something you truly appreciate.

The object of your appreciation could be something different every day, or it could be the same for weeks! The beauty of this basic meditation is that it brings us to the core of our being within a few minutes and raises our energetic vibration. Try doing a daily practice of just a few minutes when you wake up or before you go to sleep, accompanied by some very calming Sacred Sounds.

This is a practice. Be gentle and loving with yourself as you *learn to remember* to breathe, focus on your heart, and feel appreciation in challenging situations. A heart filled with compassion sends out a frequency to your whole body that brings health to all your organs and systems, slowly and safely, opening you up to all the gifts your essence has for you. I also invite you to observe if those around you become calmer.

Imagine

Another helpful and power practice is to feel yourself in a state of coherence as you imagine a difficult situation in the future. In your meditative practice you might even ask your Higher Self for an image that symbolizes your heart and brain connection.

In this way your coherent emotional responses help form new neural pathways and new patterns in your brain, along with the secretion of healthy hormones.

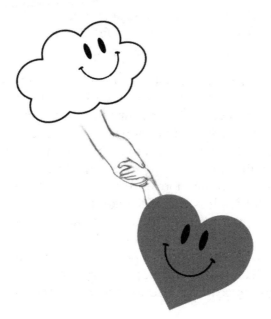

Heart and Head Connected.
December 2015. Created by Marianne Green.

Our brains do not know the difference between an image and reality. Dr. Joe Dispenza does amazing work in this area, based on the Hebbian Law: Nerve cells that fire together, wire together. Nerve cells that no longer fire together, no longer wire together. (I would say that the files are eliminated.) I myself have practiced just looking at an image (like this very simple one of the brain and the heart holding hands, which I am offering as an example until you are motivated to come up with your own!). I even put images on my computer desktop. When I am feeling ill at ease about a situation, I look at the image, go into my heart, and breathe until I feel calm, feeling the vibration of all the nuances that the image represents.

Images and sounds are vibrations—multi dimensional messages—the language of light. They are gifts from the Creator, which communicate with our physical and subtle fields.

I would like to share the most powerful tool that I have recently learned from my close connection with Inelia Benz, who has a myriad of practical tools on her website.

> *At the end of a process or clearing,*
> *ask that the situation be infused with*
> *Source Energy: Love and Light.*

It has been a great honor for me to share with you some of my favorite tools that I've practiced for decades. As a holistic inner peace activist, I know that everything is connected and all the practices that I have introduced, in combination with other practices in this beautiful book, will be the source of gentle and loving support to you, not only in this particular time challenge, but also in all your life pathways to becoming more and more the Essential Being of your soul's evolution. It is with deep compassion and reverence that I acknowledge each and every one of us as we awaken to the miracle of a mystery so grand and so beyond our human understanding. We are infused with the power of this mystery, and it is our courage that enables us to open ourselves to its wonders, and trust the guidance that is within each and every one of us, in our hearts.

Marianne Green is a musician, composer, inner peace activist, teacher, and specialist in Sound Healing. By using overtone instruments with intention and imagery, she enables people in private and group sessions, classes, workshops, and concerts to experience the transformational power of Healing Sounds. Contact Marianne at: www.sphericalimprovisations.com.

* * *

References and websites

Dr. Joe Dispenza: www.drjoedispenza.com

Eckhardt Tolle: www.eckharttolle.com

HeartMath® Institute: www.heartmath.org

Hemi-Sync: www.hemi-sync.com

John Beaulieu: www.biosonics.com

CD Soul's Garden: www.sphericalimprovisations.com/souls-gardencd.htm

Jonathan Goldman: www.healingsounds.com

Vibrational Energy Fields: The Chakra Handbook by Shalila Sharamon

34

Water Therapy

Soaking in water has been used for thousands of years as a way to heal, rejuvenate, and purify the mind, body, and spirit. It can improve sleep, boost the immune system, encourage the release of toxins, and relieve muscle aches and stiff joints. Learn which essential oils work particularly well in water, and specific ways to use water as a therapy for yourself and your care partner.

"Everything is a miracle. It is a miracle that one does not dissolve in one's bath like a lump of sugar."
–Pablo Picasso

Healing with Water Therapy

By **Laraine Pounds**, RN MSN BSN, CMT

The use of water for healing is called *hydrotherapy*. It has been used in many cultures for thousands of years, and steam bathing is one of the oldest methods. The Romans adopted steam bathing from the Greeks, and then added scented massage and exercise to their health regimens. In Rome, the acronym S P A often appeared on the walls of the steam room, which stood for solus por aqua, *healing through water*. Our modern day word *spa* was derived from this phrase. The Turkish steam bath, known as *hamam,* has survived as a tradition for thousands of years and is still in use today. In Russia, steam bathing is known as *banja*. Native Americans use a sweat lodge for purification and vision questing and Mexican Indians use natural mineral hot springs for healing their sick.

Commercial steam baths began to appear at health resorts in the 1960's. The design of steam showers have greatly improved over the last ten years and can be easily installed in almost any bathroom, providing a home-based spa environment. Included in the steam shower system are an efficient steam generator, a control system, and a steam-tight cabinet to prevent steam from escaping into the room. These self-contained units come in a variety of designs and sizes for individual family needs. Most steam showers have a convenient port for the addition of essential oils that vaporize with the steam in an aerosol mist, enhancing the health benefits of the steam shower.

Daily aromatic steam showering can become a treasured time of the day to relax, detoxify, and bond with your care partner. Explore the benefits of steam showering with essential oils for yourself.

Benefits of aromatic steam bathing

- Reduces stress
- Helps improve sleep
- Boosts the immune system
- Increases lymph system cleansing
- Stimulates blood circulation
- Encourages the release of accumulated toxins
- Alleviates respiratory congestion
- Supports the health and vibrancy of the skin
- Relieves muscle aches and stiff joints

Stress reduction

Cynthia Dorsey, PhD, the director of the Sleep Research program at McLean Hospital in Belmont, Massachusetts, found that thirty minute steam baths taken 1 1/2 to 2 hours before bedtime improved sleep in female insomniacs by approximately ten percent. Robert Ornstein, PhD and David Sobel, MD presented scientific evidence in their book *Health Pleasures* (Perseus Books, 1989) that positive attitudes and sensory pleasures support wellness and, in particular, the helpful effect of aromatics on stress and depression.

Adding aromatic essential oils to a relaxing bath is an added gesture of self-care. There are so many wonderful fragrances to choose from, such as marjoram, clary sage, and chamomile. In general, add six to eight drops of oil per bath or eight to ten drops if the bather is ill with a cold or flu. Avoid citrus and spices in hot baths due to their inherent content of citrals, which can be irritating to sensitive skin.

A dispersant agent helps the essential oils disperse into the water. Without a dispersant the oils float on top of the water. The fat in milk, cream, and vegetable oils such as coconut, helps to mix the oils with the water. Use equal parts of the dispersant with the oils, i.e. six drops of oil plus six drops of coconut oil.

How to make a refreshing bath blend

- **Relaxing Bath Blend.** Add a total of forty drops to two cups of Epsom salts, and use approximately ¼ cup for each bath. Geranium-ten drops, Rosemary- ten drops, Lavender- ten drops, Juniper-five drops, Lemongrass-five drops. Note: Salts are drying to the skin, so it's important to use a skin lotion after bathing.

- **Foot Bath.** Add two to four drops of essential oils in a small tub of water. Aromatherapy footbaths can help agitated patients calm down and rest. Soak feet for ten minutes or as tolerated. Apply a relaxing aromatherapy lotion afterwards, if tolerated.

Immune boosting

The antibacterial and antiviral properties of Tea Tree, Eucalyptus, Pine, and Niaouli oils (Melaleuca) are useful for flu and sinusitis, as well as general strengthening of the immune system. Steam inhalation directs the essential oil vapor directly to the respiratory tract where it comes in direct contact with flu germs and other respiratory irritants. Congested respiratory passages (sinuses, the bronchial tubes, and alveoli in the lungs) are opened by steam, which can provide relief from colds and other minor respiratory complaints.

Steam helps the body release toxins and cellular waste materials from the capillaries. It is reported that the sweating that occurs during a fifteen minute sauna or steam shower can flush out heavy metals such as copper, lead, zinc, and mercury. It normally takes the kidneys twenty-four hours to excrete these environmental pollutants. Sweat also helps release lactic acid from sports exertion that can cause fatigue and muscle stiffness. Steam baths provide an easy way for caregivers to strengthen an immune system that might be compromised due to stress.

Methods incorporated in Hydrotherapy:

1. Bath

2. Compress

3. Foot or hand bath/soak

4. Hot water bottle

5. Ice pack

6. Jacuzzi

7. Shower

8. Sitz bath

9. Steam bath

The following guidelines are adapted from *Aromatherapy: A Lifetime Guide to Healing with Essential Oils* by Valerie Cooksley (Prentice Hall, 1996).

Hot Bath	99 – 108 degree F	Up to twenty minutes
Warm Bath	97 – 101 degrees F	Twenty minutes to an hour
Tepid Bath	92 – 97 degrees F	Up to one hour
Cold Bath	59 – 68 degrees F	A few seconds usually in a shower

Precautions

It is best not to use hydrotherapy within an hour of eating, and do not exceed fifteen to twenty minutes at a time. Steaming should be followed by a cooling-off period before resuming a steaming session. Individuals who have low blood pressure, are elderly, obese, have heart problems, or a medical condition, should check with their health care practitioner before using extreme temperatures. Discontinue a steam session if you become dizzy or faint, or experience skin sensitivity. Rehydrate with water after steaming and apply a natural lotion or aromatic body oil to replenish the skin's naturally occurring protective mantle.

* * *

Laraine Pounds, *RN MSN BSN, CMT provides professional consulta-tion and education for healthy institutions to support the implementation of aromatherapy programs. She can be reached at:* <u>larainekp@gmail.com</u> *and via:* <u>www.Aroma-RN.com</u> *and* <u>ResourcesforLivingWell.com</u>.

Tips for Bathing the Alzheimer's Patient

Morris was a cleanliness fanatic. Before he began losing his memory, during the summer he'd take three showers a day and think nothing of it. But he, like many people with mid-to late-stage Alzheimer's disease, couldn't remember how to wash his hair or wash his body parts. Some Alzheimer's patients are embarrassed to undress in front of anyone, even if that person is their spouse. Some people get cold easily and others become afraid of the water.

Health care professionals recommend that seniors, especially those living in an assisted living facility, get showered or bathed at least twice a week. It's important to maintain a personal hygiene routine in order to reduce the possibility of urinary tract infection and to maintain healthy skin.

Bathing someone with dementia can get tricky. Here are some helpful recommendations that will help you both stay calm and feel refreshed afterwards.

- Safety first! Buy a shower seat at a medical supply store so your care partner can sit down. This eliminates fear of falling. Install a hand bar to grab onto, and a hand-held showerhead with a long hose and adjustable height. If necessary, install a shower ramp if your care partner has difficulty moving in and out of the shower.
- Keep the room brightly lit and open the curtain and shade.
- Make bathing fun. Propose this: "Let's both get spruced up and have a tea party," or "Let's both get cleaned up and then we'll go out for lunch (or dinner)."

- Spritz the bathroom with a relaxing essential oil such as chamomile, lavender, clary sage, marjoram, or spikenard.

- Make sure the bathroom is warm and not chilly.

- If you can, splurge on a towel warmer. There's nothing like getting wrapped inside a warm, terry cloth towel or robe. Towel warmers start at about one hundred and fifty-five dollars. You can also put pajamas in the dryer and have them ready to slip into. Delightful!

- Put on some relaxing classical or New Age music.

- Find a shampoo and soap fragrance that your care partner especially likes.

- Give verbal cues so there are no surprises. "I'm going to wash your hair now. Keep your eyes closed," etc.

- If privacy and modesty are major issues, hire a skilled person of the same sex from an accredited agency to bathe your care partner.

- Use a powder shampoo and sponge baths when necessary.

- Try to maintain a sense of humor and remember, "This too shall pass."

35

Yoga

If you've ever wanted to try yoga but were embarrassed to go to a class, now is your chance. Yoga therapist Reverend Sharon Shanthi Behl has worked with dementia patients and their care partners and has witnessed excellent results. Here she provides yoga postures that anyone can do and ways to create a quiet space, along with the benefits of yoga and chanting.

"Yoga does not just change the way we see things,
it transforms the person who sees."
–B.K.S. Iyengar, *Light on Life*

By Reverend **Sharon Shanthi Behl**, MA, LPC, E-RYT-500©

Historians date yogic teaching to more than five thousand years ago. There is a vast reservoir of both written information and verbal teachings that have been handed down from teacher to student in unbroken lineages across generations. My spiritual lineage, brought from India to the United States in the 1970's by Sri Swami Satchidananda, combines various methods of yoga including chanting, eye exercises, breath practices, guided deep relaxation (called *yoga nidra*), meditation, selfless service, and a deep commitment to the inclusive acceptance of all spiritual paths. If you are of a certain age, you might remember that Swami Satchidananda led the Woodstock nation in the chanting of the sacred Sanskrit sound "Om" during the festival's opening ceremonies.

In the early 1920's in the United States the word *yoga* conjured up a picture of turbaned East Indian men in pretzel-shaped contortions performing for photographers from *Life Magazine*. And for many decades afterwards, yoga was viewed primarily with suspicion. As a child, I remember how the word yoga was often mistaken for the word yogurt. Fast forward to today and we see an explosion of yoga images and references in popular culture. Photos of people doing yoga poses are as ubiquitous as Starbucks cafes. Open a random magazine and you are likely to see a photo of a young, lithe, leotard-clad woman, arms outstretched at shoulder height, standing in warrior pose on a purple mat touting the benefits of diet soda, a hotel chain, or even a car!

Needless to say, this popularity has its downside. With the commercialism of yoga, and the widespread images in magazine advertising, television and movies, one of the unfortunate results is that many older, bigger, stiff-jointed Americans cannot imagine themselves practicing yoga, even in their wildest dreams.

If you have that concern, here's some good news. In the process of yoga becoming mainstream, it has also been adapted for people of practically every age, size, shape, and physical or mental condition. Just a quick search of the word yoga on the internet today reveals 89,600,000 results. Type in Alzheimer's disease + Yoga and you see more than 2,000,000 citations! Although there is no lack of information out there, *caveat emptor*. If you want to explore yoga more deeply, use common sense and, even better, consult a credentialed or otherwise reputable teacher. There are accessible yogic practices for everybody!

My life is already too complicated!

Let me tell you something. It may sound irrational, but in my experience, it is a totally predicable phenomenon. When I practice yoga first thing in the morning for at least fifteen minutes before I start work, I absolutely have more time in my day. I accomplish more tasks and the time between events seems more spacious. This is unrelated to what time I wake up, the number of deadlines looming over my head, or the state of my appointment calendar. My mood is more even. I experience set-backs, jammed copiers, words that will not form on the page, and people who cut me off in traffic with much less drama. I am more fully engaged with my day and yet it is easier to cultivate a more peaceful sense of detachment from stressors. I feel a wider sense of compassion and patience with those whose viewpoint is, let's say, *different* than mine.

The positive effects are also evident when a true crisis emerges. I am often called upon for my calming presence to deal with someone who is angry or irrational. I attribute this phenomenon to the practice of yoga. I have noticed this effect for years. I also notice the waves of frustration, impatience, judgment, and anxiety swelling within me when I have neglected my practice for even two or three days. I encourage you to see how yoga can show up in your own life.

Now, I'd like to introduce you to Al and Jean and how they engaged in the practice of yoga.

Practicing Yoga Together in the Last Days of Life

On a brilliant autumn morning, Al and Jean (*names changed*) hesitantly entered the hospital classroom where our first yoga class was being held. They were smartly dressed in new matching navy blue sweat pants and sweatshirts. Al was wheeling a portable oxygen tank alongside his bent, but still imposingly tall frame. He wore a puzzled look and did not speak when I welcomed them. Jean quickly and somewhat anxiously explained their situation. She was hoping they could attend class together. Last month, Al had been diagnosed with Alzheimer's disease.

Jean shared that getting the diagnosis was actually a relief. It explained many of the odd behaviors her husband of thirty-five years had been exhibiting over the past year. For example, just that morning, he became very anxious as Jean was driving them to class. He was convinced that the car they were in belonged to someone else and he was afraid of being arrested. She was, as she put it, at her wit's end and feeling desperate. Years ago she had taken a yoga class at her local recreational center and she thought that maybe a therapeutic yoga class could bring Al the sense of peace she had experienced back then. A friend had also mentioned that yoga was good for stress management and that Jean might benefit because of the stress of being a full-time caregiver.

Jean was, understandably, concerned about her husband becoming upset during class or wandering away. But once class began it was Jean, not Al, who took longer to settle down. She had a difficult time staying focused and I observed her sneaking a look at her husband in the middle of a pose. After some time, when she was assured that he was safe and quietly going along with the instructions, she seemed to attune more deeply to her own body and her facial tension began to melt.

Al and Jean showed up for class once a week for two and a half months, before Al suddenly passed away from complications of a chronic respiratory illness. During the weeks they attended, I could see Jean's body beginning to relax. Although she was unable to comfortably get from sitting on the floor to standing, she progressed to standing easily without assistance. Jean reported that her back stopped hurting, even after giving Al his bath; an activity that previously caused her lower back muscles to knot up with tension. Jean also shared that she was more patient with Al's pacing and found that she did not feel like screaming at him quite as often. In fact, she confided that she started to be much more playful and silly with Al.

This all made sense to me. When we deeply relax emotionally and physically we can experience stressful situations with some humor and an appreciation of the absurdities that life brings us. We can instead, quite literally, laugh with compassion toward others and ourselves when our hearts are breaking.

Yoga postures for you to try at home

Here's a posture that I taught in every class. Jean particularly liked to do this while standing in the grocery line. This is called mountain pose or *tadasana*.

1. *Stand with your feet parallel and a few inches apart. Imagine the sole of each foot as a rectangle and let your weight be equally distributed across each of the four corners.*

2. *Allow the knees to soften and feel a sense of lengthening up the legs. Begin lifting up the front of the body. Lift the ribcage away from the pelvis and hips and feel a sense of widening and opening across the center of the chest (known as the heart center).*

3. *Lift the shoulders up towards the ears, roll them back behind you giving a good squeeze as if you could touch the shoulder blades together, and then roll the shoulders down away from the ears.*

Repeat three to four times and then repeat rolling in the opposite direction.

4. *Bring the shoulders to stillness, allowing them to continue dropping away from the ears and relax the arms and hands heavily by your sides as if you are holding a gallon of water in each hand.*

5. *Finally, gently press the crown of your head up to the sky, even while you press your feet into the earth below. Stand in this manner, tall as a mountain, and breathe naturally for three to five minutes (or as long as it takes you to move to the front of the check-out line!)*

Mountain pose brings with it a bodily-felt sense of the qualities of a mountain. It helps one cultivate patience and steadiness in the midst of the emotional storms of life.

You must take excellent care of yourself

You have probably heard people tell you that you must take care of yourself when you are the caregiver. You probably know something about "burn-out" and compassion fatigue, and perhaps you picked up this book as prevention. On the other hand, you may already feel burnt to a crisp.

According to a report published by the *UCLA Newsroom*, the incidence and prevalence of clinical depression in family dementia caregivers approaches fifty percent. Dr. Helen Lavretsky, professor of psychiatry at the University of California at Los Angeles (UCLA) Semel Institute for Neuroscience and Human Behavior, has noted that many caregivers tend to be older themselves, leading to what Lavretsky has termed an "impaired resilience" to stress and an increased rate of cardiovascular disease and mortality. To investigate, she and her colleagues conducted a study where caregivers were taught a twelve-minute chanting practice. The participants in the study practiced every day for eight weeks. Their findings suggest that simple daily practice can lead to improved cognitive functioning and lower levels of depression for caregivers. The researchers found that "…our study suggests a simple, low-cost yoga program can enhance coping and quality of life for the caregivers."

Studies such as these are becoming more common, and medical science is confirming what practitioners of yoga have known all along. The practice of yoga *asana*, *pranayama*, chanting, and meditation profoundly benefits the mental health of the practitioner.

When we are burned out, we think we can feel better by doing more. Our mind can be mistakenly convinced that we can solve a problem with the same thinking that created the problem in the first place. We soldier on as if we can handle everything ourselves, instead of opening up to the comfort and support of others. Often we must learn to "try softer," rather than harder, and "let go" rather than grasp more firmly. Instead, we must listen to our heart's inner promptings. The wisdom of yoga teaches us the value of non-doing, being still, and sitting with equanimity with whatever life presents.

The caregiving staff at *Grandma's Cottage* reported the benefits that yoga class had on themselves and their residents. This story illustrates how caregivers at a facility increased their consciousness of *saucha* (purity) and *ahimsa* (non-violence) and improved their own sense of well-being, along with that of their residents. The names of the people and the agency have been changed.

Angelique Stokes worked as a head nurse at *Grandma's Cottage*, a clean and pleasantly furnished memory-care facility that provided twenty-four hour care. Angelique contacted me looking for someone to teach yoga to their staff. *Grandma's Cottage* was professionally run and it was clear that management wanted to invest in the care of their staff in order to better serve their residents. It was also obvious that staff members were in danger of compassion fatigue or burn-out.

After our first class, I entered the living room where many of the residents sat in a semi-circle and watched television after breakfast. The screams of a woman being pursued by a hideous groaning monster emanated from the TV set and rang throughout the building. My experience was visceral and immediate as muscles tightened, adrenaline coursed through my body, my field of vision narrowed, and my entire system kicked into the kind of response our bodies are wired to do when faced with real and immediate danger. After a brief moment, my senses confirmed that I was not at risk of being eaten by a large wild animal. Yet, for many minutes afterward, my shoulders remained tight and I could feel the beginnings of a slight headache. Most of the residents could not voluntarily leave the room and appeared to be in various states of discomfort. Some had their eyes closed, but I could see them startle each time the woman screamed. One resident sat in her wheelchair with her torso twisted away from the TV screen and stared at the wall. Not one person appeared to be enjoying this horror film.

In contrast, staff members were busy with the post-breakfast chores and moved in and out of the room talking amongst themselves. They appeared oblivious to what was taking place with the residents. I gently approached Angelique who said she could see nothing wrong with leaving this kind of movie on. She explained it was a classic horror movie from the residents' childhood years, and thought most of them enjoyed it. She conceded that it was a little loud, however, and she would turn it down if it bothered me. It felt unskillful for me to continue to push my point, but soon another opportunity presented itself.

A few weeks later, Angelique took me aside to share this story. The previous week in yoga class, she experienced the deepest sense of relaxation she had felt in a long time. "I felt the way I used to feel as a young child floating in the pool. I had no fear or tension and felt absolutely safe," she said. "After yoga class, I passed the TV on the way to the kitchen and felt like a wall of water smacked me down. There was a program on where two people were insulting each other and every few seconds the laugh track came on. Well, I used to think this show was funny, but this time when I heard the laugh track it was like being punched in the stomach. What's going on here?"

We had a great conversation about how our environment affects every level of our being. I introduced Angelique to the yogic concepts of *saucha* (purity) and *ahimsa* (non-violence). We talked about the effects of negativity and the opposite effect when one surrounds oneself with *sattvic* (balanced) elements, such as peaceful uplifting sounds, beautiful colors and images, pleasant smells, joyful people, and healthy and delicious food and drink. Finally, we talked about the effects a steady stream of TV, movies, magazines, radio, and other media has on us, and sadly laughed at the kinds of messages we are subjected to during an average day. Basically, advertising is designed to make us feel incomplete or incompetent unless we buy the product that is being sold.

At this point, Angelique realized how the residents were being affected by some of the staff choices of entertainment. It became clear to her that it could be a win-win situation for staff and the residents if the sounds and sights of the day were more peaceful, joyful, and uplifting. Indeed, as the weeks went by, she happily reported that mornings went more smoothly when she instructed staff to avoid horror movies and programs with emotionally jarring material, and find something like "Animal Planet" or the "Cooking Channel." Better still, they used music more frequently and became aware of the tone of their voices when speaking to each other and the residents.

An easy way to increase your sense of peace

1. *Take several deep breaths and look around your immediate environment.*

2. *Identify three things that strike you as harsh, negative, or stress inducing. It could be the annoying hum of an appliance, a scary photo on a book jacket, the lingering odor of an overripe banana, or the scratchiness of a cheap blanket.*

3. *Then identify three things that are beautiful, calming, inspiring, or relaxing; perhaps a bowl of dried lavender petals, the sight of golden sunbeams across a clean carpet, the feel of a smooth seashell, or the sound of soothing classical music.*

4. *Notice the effect each thing has on your breathing and your emotions. Right now, make one change in your environment that will reduce your sense of unease and increase your sense of peace.*

Yoga teaches us through experience to pay attention to the world around us. It sensitizes us to how things affect us and how we affect others. In practical terms, the more that *Grandma's* staff provided calm, peaceful, and uplifting stimuli to the residents, the greater the sense of well-being for the staff and residents.

Chanting

You might be familiar with the use of chanting sacred sounds in yoga practice. One result of chanting is that it helps to replace the negativity that flows through our minds on a daily basis. Stop and think for a moment. When you talk to yourself, do you tend to encourage, praise, and cheer yourself on? Or do you usually berate yourself for something you did not do, or replay a conversation that went badly with a friend? In all likelihood, the words we tell ourselves do little to improve our well-being. I am fond of saying that if we talked to our friends the way we talk to ourselves, we would not have any friends!

Chanting is one way to clear our minds, to counterweight the negativity we have absorbed from the world around us, and return to that relaxed and resourceful state of mind. Chanting the name of whoever or whatever you hold sacred is a powerful option, but chanting does not have to be religious. You may think of it as repeating an uplifting sound to replace the internal chatter. Like the old song says, "Accent the positive, eliminate the negative."

Take a moment to clear your mind and give yourself a "mental shower" using the techniques of chanting. In yoga we repeat Sanskrit terms such as "Om" or various names for God. In my tradition we use repetition of sacred Sanskrit words in a manner that has been used for thousands of years. You can pick a prayer from your own religious tradition, or you may pick a more common word that has positive and peaceful vibrations such as "love" or "peace." You can also personalize this practice by chanting the names of your beloved family or friends. Finally, you may choose a phrase that holds meaning for you such as "May all my actions be born of compassion," or "For the highest good of all concerned," or "Let go, let God." It is best to pick one and stick with it for a few months rather than switching it up.

At first, you may wish to count your repetitions to keep your mind focused by using a rosary or a 108-bead necklace called a *mala*. Each bead helps to hold your count and keep your attention as you slide the beads between your fingers. Another way is to set a timer and simply set a goal of a certain number of minutes instead of repetitions. Starting with three minutes, you can work your way up to thirty minutes.

Take a moment to center and breathe deeply. Let nothing distract you as you silently repeat your special word or phrase. Set a goal of eighteen repetitions to start and work your way up to one hundred and eight or more, if you wish.

Finding a sense of peace

Yoga offers many doorways through which we can find our own true nature of peace. The regular practice of any of the above yogic techniques will reveal benefits for every level of being: physical, energetic, mental, emotional, and spiritual. May you find a useful practice that can carry you through the difficult challenges of caring for your loved one. My wish for you is twofold: may you find wellness in the support of others, and may you feel the limitless peace that can be found within. *Namaste* (The light and wisdom in me honors the light and wisdom in you).

* * *

*Reverend **Sharon Shanthi Behl**, MA, LPC, E-RYT-500©, is ordained and credentialed as a teacher through Integral Yoga, founded by Sri Swami Satchidananda. Shanthi is a founding Board member of Yoga Alliance, Board Emeritus of Yoga Teachers of Colorado and former Advisory Board member of Rocky Mountain Institute of Yoga and Ayurveda. Shanthi provides yoga instruction to hospice patients and their caregivers by integrating contemporary Western psychology with yoga's profound wisdom. She can be reached at:* peacepug2@hotmail.com.

* * *

References

Lavretsky, H., Epel, E. S., Siddarth, P., Nazarian, N., Cyr, N.S., Khalsa, D.S., et al. 2013. "A pilot study of yogic meditation for family dementia caregivers with depressive symptoms: effects on mental health, cognition, and telomerase activity." *International Journal of Geriatric Psychiatry.* 28(1): 57-65.

Satchidananda, Swami. *Healing From Disaster.* (Yogaville, VA: Integral Yoga Publications, 2006).

Smith, Sri Swami. 2013. "Alzheimer's Disease." *Mayo Clinic Health Letter.* www.mayoclinic.com/health/sundowning/HQ01463.

Part Four

✕

When Caregiving Ends

36

Courage, Strength, and Valor

Rabbi Peter J. Rubinstein, rabbi emeritus of the Central Synagogue in New York City, gave a sermon on October 5, 2005, in which he spoke about how the Jewish holidays of Rosh Hashanah and Yom Kippur remind us of the passing of years, of how quickly even the last year has gone. The following is an excerpt from his talk -

"And to live well is to love well."

"The vector of life is indisputable. We are born and we get older. At some point we realize that we're closer to the end than the beginning of life. Each day's experiences become wisdom for the next. Time rolls by at a breathless tempo. We are intent in savoring each moment.

"Then, rather unexpectedly, there comes the juncture for which we are completely untrained, when we become caregivers to our own parents. It is on the minds of many of us. Without instruction from our parents about what they want and totally unprepared for the emotional impact, we become parents to our parents. We attempt to maintain their dignity and self-esteem even when their diminishing physical abilities become a critical affront to their independence and pride. Our parents suffer because they don't want to be a burden on us. We want them to know that we are pleased to do for them a small part of what they did for us when we were young. And then suddenly it dawns on us that the time will come when we, like our parents, will need the care of others.

"We understand that it is tough to be old. It is painful to mourn a spouse or lose friends or wait for visits from family who are understandably busy in their own lives. It is difficult to live by ourselves at the end of life, to be nursed by caregivers or in a residence we know to be our last.

"Being old takes remarkable courage and I'm awed by the valor of all who bravely face mortality and who, in the words of Rabbi Zalman Schachter-Shalomi 'use the information of long life to gain wisdom.' It takes enormous strength and it is to be honored.

There is timeless wisdom in our tradition on how to live well at every age. This is what we learn: Anticipate each day with hope. Love. Be holy."

Rabbi Rubinstein concluded his sermon with a beautiful anecdote about a member of his congregation who would often visit her memory-impaired mother. "Her mother would ask, 'Please, tell me about my life.' The daughter cogently and patiently recounted the stories she remembered and heard from her mother: when her mother was young, when her mother came to this country, when her mother married. Then she added her own recollections of her mother from her own childhood and teen-age years and beyond. When she finished the narrative her mother, after a moment, reflected, 'It was a good life, wasn't it?'"

* * *

*Rabbi **Peter J. Rubinstein** joined Central Synagogue as senior rabbi in 1991. Under his leadership and vision, Rabbi Rubinstein revitalized the congregation in all areas including liturgy, education, and organizational structure, bringing Central Synagogue into the twenty-first century. In his current role as rabbi emeritus – along with being an active member of the congregation – Rabbi Rubinstein is a member of the Melton teaching team and Co-President of the U.S. Board of the Tony Blair Faith Foundation. He oversees the Bronfman Center for Jewish Life as the 92Y's Director of Jewish Community and sits on the board of the Tony Blair Faith Foundation. He is recognized as a leader in the changing face of the Jewish community and was ranked number three in Newsweek's 2012 list of "America's 50 Most Influential Rabbis." He has been on the list since its inception.*

His writing has been included in several books including, Our Rabbis Taught *(1990),* How Can I Find God *(1997),* Restoring Faith *(2001), and* Shine by Star Jones *(2006). Reach Rabbi Rubinstein at:* <u>clergy@ censyn.org</u>.

37

Living With Hope

Caregiving for a person with dementia is one of the most difficult things anyone will ever have to do. The pain and suffering is intense, but the rewards are plenty. Even though the person you are caring for cannot express gratitude, on some level they know and appreciate your sacrifice. They are eternally indebted to you. As Lou Gehrig said in his farewell speech, "When you have a wife (caregiver) who has been a tower of strength and shown more courage than you dreamed exists — that's the finest I know. So I close in saying that I might have been given a bad break, but I've got an awful lot to live for."

I heard time and time again from Morris's friends and other caregivers about how much he loved and appreciated me. His last words to me were, "I love you." Even though he couldn't thank me for taking care of him, I knew . . . I just knew . . . and I'm so glad I was able to fulfill my promise to care for him up until the end.

Kim Mooney, the Board President of Conversations on Death, and Director of Community Education for Tru Community Care, Colorado's first hospice, has said that as caregivers "the sacrifices you made changed the course of your life. As you once again look at finding a new course, you will over time grieve your loved one and what you let go of or stored away. You will also begin to discover the things you learned from giving so much. As you recognize and honor what you did, it will begin to shape the meaning of your life now. Whatever the challenges ahead in rebuilding, that understanding can give you the strength, commitment, and satisfaction to make your life more meaningful than ever."

So, what's next? Stop, take a deep breath, and think about your journey: where you came from, what you did, and how you feel. When Morris's final health crisis was over and after I buried him, I realized that I hadn't fully breathed for years and that my body was strangled with tension and fatigue. I had meditated, eaten fairly well (besides the times I was too tired to cook and made a dinner out of popcorn and ice cream), danced, exercised, and practiced yoga. All these things helped keep me calm, and brought me back to my "self." But being on call for years took its toll. And after it was all over, while ensnared in the tentacles of grieving, I felt relief. Relief that I wouldn't feel the pain of watching Morris lose yet another function. Relief that I wouldn't have to fill another prescription or talk to a physician about my husband's condition. Relief that I didn't have to travel the fifteen miles to visit him in the memory care home, where I'd inevitably get depressed. Relief that I could stay home and not have an obligation other than caring for myself.

And yet, the final letting go of my role as caregiver was uncomfortable and felt strangely similar to sending my children out into the world. How would I define myself if I were no longer a caregiver? How would I fill up the time I had spent caring for my husband for an entire decade, one fifth of my life? Creating a new identity takes time, practice, and patience. And we are told by grief counselors to not rush things. Do not make a major change in your life, such as moving out of the house you've lived in for years, or to another state. But day-by-day, it's okay to acknowledge that we are not the same person who, along with our loved one, heard the doctor's dreaded words: "You have dementia, most likely of the Alzheimer's type."

As caregivers we take a journey through fire and ice and land on solid ground surrounded by calm waters. Then it's time to swim to shore and get our bearings. Many ways to help you get there have been discussed in the previous pages and there are still more out there like learning to play an instrument, volunteering at a homeless shelter or joining a book club. Be patient, be kind to yourself, and set out to discover different activities, small and large, that ease you to calmer waters.

My journey to calmer waters

My husband's illness changed the course of my family's lives in ways that were unexpected, devastating, and empowering. I developed into a strong matriarch and quickly learned how to take charge of my husband's care, family business, and my children, without the help of my partner. And not having a partner, with whom I would typically make important decisions, was one of the hardest things of all about being a partner to someone with Alzheimer's disease. Deciding where and when to place Morris in a memory care home, figuring out how to finance it, and deciding when to enlist the help of hospice were the kinds of decisions I would have discussed with my husband.

I became a compassionate caregiver, not just for Morris, but for other residents of the memory care home where he lived the last two years of his life. I went through a lot—as all caregivers do—but I've come through. I've recreated my life, and have learned to look forward with hope, wonder, delight, and inspiration after giving so much of myself to the person I vowed to spend my life with.

There are days that go by without my thinking about Morris, and once in a while I burst out crying because I can't believe that he is gone. It's still hard for me to look at family photos because our family was happy, and a link is missing. I know for my children the hardest thing is that their own children are growing up without knowing their grandfather, who would have loved to be a part of their lives. But we keep his memory alive by showing his picture to them, remembering his beautiful smile and contagious laughter, and by striving to emulate his sweetness. We will always miss him, but our happy memories fill in the gaps, and we honor him every year on his yahrzeit, the anniversary of a Jewish loved one's death.

It seems like yesterday that I was a college student wearing my lace-up moccasins, patched jeans and sky blue sweatshirt when I first heard Morris lecture about how Transcendental Meditation can help us to live more fulfilled and happier lives. He was my teacher then, and he continues to teach me now about compassion, devotion, and the deeper meaning of life.

I have a new love in my life and grandchildren to enjoy and cherish. I feel good and I am happy! As my beloved teacher Sri Sai Kaleshwar Swami always said, "Life is short, make it sweet." I will and I do. And I encourage you to do the same.

Eulogy of Morris Cohn

Moshe ben Noam haCohen u'Devorah

September 2, 2010

by Rabbi **Marc Soloway**

"One week from today, Jews all over the world will be celebrating Rosh Hashanah, the Jewish new year. The characteristic qualities of the time leading up to the High Holidays, the month of Elul, are about introspection, spiritual intimacy, and seeking to heal and repair any hurt in our relationships. How appropriate for Morris Cohn, who was a deeply spiritual man, a practitioner and teacher of meditation, and a person who took all of his personal relationships very seriously and with great integrity. Barbra shared with me that if Morris ever felt that he had even remotely hurt someone, he would feel it very deeply and would always get on the phone and be willing to apologize. Morris was a wonderful teacher in so many ways, including of course, Transcendental Meditation, teaching over a thousand people to meditate, and he continues to teach us. Perhaps he is teaching us to make sure that we too reach out to those in our lives that we may have hurt and that we have the integrity and compassion to heal.

In the Vedic tradition, which was so important to Morris, today is marked as the birthday of Krishna who is the human embodiment of loving kindness and compassion. How perfect for Morris whose essence was of pure love, compassion, and kindness. Even though Morris had Alzheimer's since before I met him, I still feel blessed to have known him and in my visits, I would experience the great love of this man, shining from his gentle soul, transcending the confusion of his mind and the increasing weakness of his body. I always enjoyed my visits with Morris, who would always greet me so warmly and sometimes he would just repeat the names of those he loved with a sense of concern and trust that they were all doing alright. "Barbra's doing okay I guess, and there's Hillary and Daniel, Ari and Ronit, and Bobette." Over and over he would say these names as if they were a mantra.

Morris was a loving husband to Barbra and a great father, as well as a businessman, teacher, spiritual healer, and a loyal friend to so many. He didn't quite belong in his generation with his hippy idealism, his adventurous spirit, and his love of rock music. Morris also had an amazing memory for facts, especially history that he loved. He was a great outdoorsman and passionate about gardening and growing. In some ways he was quite complex, and there is a sad irony to the fact that the dreadful disease that took him over simplified him to his essence, even beyond the pain and frustration for him and the family. Even when words were hard to find, Morris could always communicate love and compassion for everyone, whoever it was. Barbra said that he was so intensely spiritual earlier in life that he would become enraptured and cry from the depths of his huge, open heart.

There is no doubt that the disease caused him, and all his family, torment and suffering. On Tuesday morning, however, as he made his transition to the ultimate embrace of all life, he was so at peace. Sad as this loss is, there was something perfect, almost blissful at the very end and, as Barbra noticed, he looked very young, as if he had released himself from an enormous burden. He looked so at peace in that moment, surrounded by Barbra, Ari, Hillary, Daniel and Ronit, whose great love gave him permission to leave his troubled mind and body and enter that realm of pure spirit, which had always been part of him.

Although Morris had not been brought up steeped in Judaism and his main spirituality certainly came from the Vedic tradition, Judaism nevertheless was very important to him. Like me, Morris was a Cohen, a member of the priestly tribe — he was like a priest. I remember how he used to enjoy coming up on the bimah (alter) during the High Holidays to join the other Cohanim for the special blessing ritual of the Birkat Cohanim, a very powerful incantation. "May God bless you and keep you. May God's face shine on you and be gracious to you. May God lift that face on you and give you peace."

In Morris' honor, I would like to invite us to join in a loving kindness meditation, based on this threefold blessing, sending the loving intention into the universe and to Morris' soul as he makes his transition into the divine embrace. May you feel safe. May you feel happy. May you feel peaceful. Please receive this blessing for yourself and send this blessing to Morris and then to all beings.

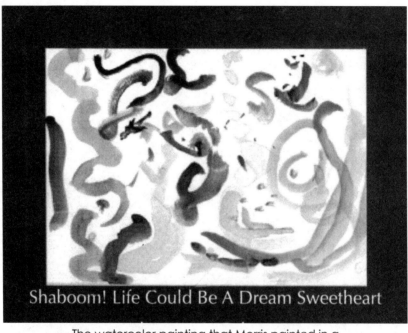

Shaboom! Life Could Be A Dream Sweetheart

The watercolor painting that Morris painted in a
Memories in the Making® workshop.

Appendix

Further Reading

- Atchley Jenny & Adele Britton. *The Hokey Pokey Is What It's All About*. LightenUp Press, 2007.

- Bauman, Edward, EdM, PhD *Recipes & Remedies For Rejuvenation*. Bauman College Press, 2005.

- Bauman, Edward, EdM, PhD *Eating for Health: Your Guide to Vitality & Optimal Health*. Bauman College Press, 2008.

- Bauman, Edward, EdM, PhD, Marx, Lizette. *Flavors of Health Cookbook*. Bauman College Press, 2012.

- Bell, Virginia & Troxel, David. *A Dignified Life: The Best Friends Approach to Alzheimer's Care*. Health Communications, 2002.

- Bryden, Christine. *Dancing with Dementia*. Jessica Kingsley Publishers, 2005.

- Bryden, Christine. *Before I Forget: How I Survived a Diagnosis of Younger-Onset* Dementia. Penguin Books Australia, 2015.

- Buber, Martin. *I and Thou*. Touchstone 1st Touchstone edition Feb. 1971.

- Coste, Joanne Koenig. *Learning to Speak Alzheimer's*. First Mariner Books, 2003.

- Dispenza, Joe. *Evolve Your Brain*. HCI, Oct. 2008.

- Douillard, John. *The 3-Season Diet* Three Rivers Press, 2000.

- Forrest, Deborah A. *Symphony of Spirits*, St. Martin's Press, 2000.

- Goldman, Connie. *The Gifts of Caregiving*. Fairview Press, 2012.

- Jacobs, C. (2010). Exploring religion and spirituality in clinical practice. *Smith College Studies in Social Work, 80*(2-3). New York: Taylor & Francis.

- Jacobs, C. (2004). Spirituality and end-of-life care practice for social workers. In Berzoff, J. & Silverman, P.R. (Eds.). *Living with dying: a textbook on end-of-life care for social work.* NY: Columbia University Press.

- Jacobs, C. (February, 2004). Spiritually-centered therapy. In Dorfman, R. & Morgan, M. (Eds.), *Paradigms of clinical social work: Focus on diversity* (Vol. 3). NY: Taylor and Francis.

- McLeod, Beth Witrogen. *Caregiving: The Spiritual Journey of Love, Loss, and Renewal.* John Wiley & Sons, 1999.

- Miller, James E. *The Caregiver's Book: Caring for Another, Caring for Yourself.* Willowgreen Publishing; Second edition (October 10, 2008).

- Ornstein, Robert, PhD and Sobel, David, MD *Health Pleasures.* Persus Books, 1989.

- Telushkin, Joseph. *Words that Hurt, Words that Heal.* William Morrow, 1998.

- Tolle, Eckhart. *The Power of Now: A Guide to Spiritual Enlightenment.* Namaste Publishing, 2004.

- Thich Nhat Hanh. Reproduced from *For a Future to Be Possible: Commentaries on the Five Wonderful Precepts* 1993 Parallax Press, 1993.

- Rando, Therese, A. *Grief, Dying and Death: Clinical Interventions for Caregivers.* Research PR Pub., 1984.

- Rando, Therese, A. *How to Go On Living When Someone You Love Dies.* Bantam, 1991.

Resources

Alzheimer's Association National Office
225 North Michigan Avenue, Floor 17, Chicago, IL 60601
24/7 Helpline: 1.800.272.3900

www.alz.org

The Alzheimer's Association offers information, a help line, and support services to people with Alzheimer's and their caregivers. Local chapters across the country offer support groups, including many that help with early-stage Alzheimer's. To find support groups in your area, call 1-800-272-3900.

Find downloadable resources at: twww.alz.org/health-care-pro-fessionals/patient-information-education-care-resources.asp.

NIH Senior Health: nihseniorhealth.gov/alzheimerscare/caregiversupport/01.html.

The Alzheimer's Disease Education and Referral (ADEAR) Center offers information on diagnosis, treatment, patient care, caregiver needs, long-term care, research, and clinical trials related to Alzheimer's. Staff can refer you to local and national resources, or you can search for information on the website. The Center, a service of the National Institute on Aging, can be reached at: 1-800-438-4380 or www.nia.nih.gov/alzheimers.

The Alzheimer's Foundation of America provides information about Alzheimer's caregiving and a list of services for people with Alzheimer's. Services include a toll-free hotline, publications, and other educational materials. Contact the Foundation at: 1-866-232-8484.

Program of All-Inclusive Care for the Elderly (PACE) is a program that combines Medicare and Medicaid benefits. It pays medical, social service, and long-term care costs for frail, low-income people age fifty-five and older. PACE permits most people who qualify to continue living at home instead of moving to a long-term care facility. The program is available only in certain areas. To find out more, visit: **PACE**.

Social Security Disability Income is for people younger than age 65 who are disabled according to the Social Security Administration's definition. You must be able to show that the person with Alzheimer's is unable to work, and that his or her condition will last at least a year or is expected to result in death. Visit: www.ssa.gov/pgm/disability.htm for details.

Social Security also has "compassionate allowances" to help people with early-onset Alzheimer's disease, mixed dementia, fronto-temporal dementia/Pick's disease, primary progressive aphasia, and other serious medical conditions get disability benefits more quickly. To find out more, call 1-800-772-1213 or visit: www.socialsecurity.gov/compassionateallowances.

The State Health Insurance Assistance Program (SHIP) is another resource for caregivers. This is a national program offered in each State that provides free counseling and advice about Medicare coverage and benefits. To contact a SHIP counselor in your State, visit: www.medicare.gov/contacts.

Help for Veterans

If the person with Alzheimer's disease is a veteran, he or she may qualify for long-term care provided by the U.S. Department of Veterans Affairs (VA). There could be a waiting list for VA nursing homes. The VA also provides some at-home care. To learn more about VA benefits, call 1-877-222-8387 or visit: www.va.gov/health.

For more information, order a print copy of **Getting Help with Caregiving** by calling 1-800-222-2225 or visiting www.nia.nih.gov/health.

Apps for Caregivers

Wandering/Tracking, GPS

"Comfort Zone Check-in Mobile" – free – mobile app allowing access to a full service offering requiring subscription/monthly fee, Alzheimer's location management program.

"GPS Tracker" free locator for family member who has an iPhone/iPad with them.

"GPS Tracking" – $3.99 – locator for family member who has an iPhone/iPad with them.

Medication Management

"RXmindme" – free – medication reminder app
"Pill Reminder" – $0.99 – maintains prescription info, schedule reminders & access info.

"MedCoach Medication" – free – medication reminder; can connect to your pharmacy.

Caregiving

"Balance for Alzheimer's Caregivers" – $0.99 – coordinate care/meds, track changes.

"Caretaker" – free – prescription/medical records, reminders.

"Capzule PHR Your Personal Health Record"- free – maintain health info on family.

"Healthspek PHR Personal Health Record" – free – maintain health info.

"Caregiver's Touch" – $4.99 – store and share medical info/appointments/financial data/more.

"Unfrazzle" – free – care coordination app, to do list, journaling.

"Lotsa Helping Hands" – free – care coordination/task coverage by volunteers/calendar/blog.

"CareZone" – free – store and share medical info/appointments/ to do list/private data.

"CareCoach" – free – collect info relating to doctor visits.

"AD Caregiver Diary" – $4.99 – record medical symptoms/behaviors and map over time.

"Skype for iPhone" – free – voice/video calls with anyone on Skype; share photos.

"Cozi" – free – shared calendar and to do/lists for an entire family or caregiving team.

"Tyze" – free – share messages, stories/updates, and photos among family or caregiving team.

Alzheimer's Information and Resources

"Balance for Alzheimer's Caregivers" – $0.99 – caregiving tools, plus research and news.

"WebMD" – free – mobile-optimized health information.

"3D Brain" – free – interactive, 3D resource on the brain; shows disorders, functionality.

Index

About the Author

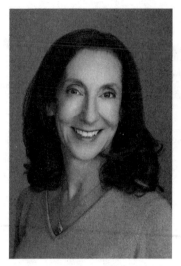

Barbra Cohn has been a professional writer for thirty-eight years, and has written hundreds of health and travel articles for national, regional and local publications. For a decade, she cared for her husband, Morris, who passed away from younger-onset Alzheimer's disease at age sixty-nine.

As president and owner of Cohn Writing Solutions, Barbra writes sales copy, newsletters and articles, and analyzes scientific studies for cosmetics and nutritional supplement companies. Her writing has appeared in AAA's *EnCompass Magazine, First for Women, Shofar, YM, Sh'ma, Delicious!, Better Nutrition, Energy Times, Inside Karate, Conscious Choice, Girls' Life* and numerous other magazines and newspapers. She is also an award-winning poet.

In addition to holding a Master's degree in professional writing, Barbra holds a BA in both English and Religious Studies and a Certificate in Nutrition from the Bauman College of Nutrition. As a nutrition educator, she offers nutritional support to caregivers, guiding them to make healthy food and lifestyle choices.

Barbra has lived in Boulder, Colorado since 1972, where she and her husband raised their two children. Her greatest pleasures include spending time with her grandchildren, dancing, meditating, traveling, and hiking in the beautiful Rocky Mountains. Email Barbra at <u>healthwriter1@gmail.com</u>; visit her blog at <u>barbracohn.com.</u>